DEVOTIONAL FOR WOMEN WITH CANCER

5-MINUTE PRAYERS & DEVOTIONS TO HELP BATTLE ISOLATION, DEEPEN YOUR CONNECTION WITH GOD, & MAINTAIN HOPE IN UNCERTAIN TIMES

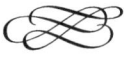

BIBLICAL TEACHINGS

FAB PUBLISHING

warriorwarriorwarriorwarri
orwarriorwarriorwarriorwa
rriorwarriorwarriorwarrior
warriorwarriorwarriorwarri
orwarriorwarriorwarriorwa
rriorwarriorwarriorwarrior

To: Lindsey
From: Mom — ~~From~~ Love

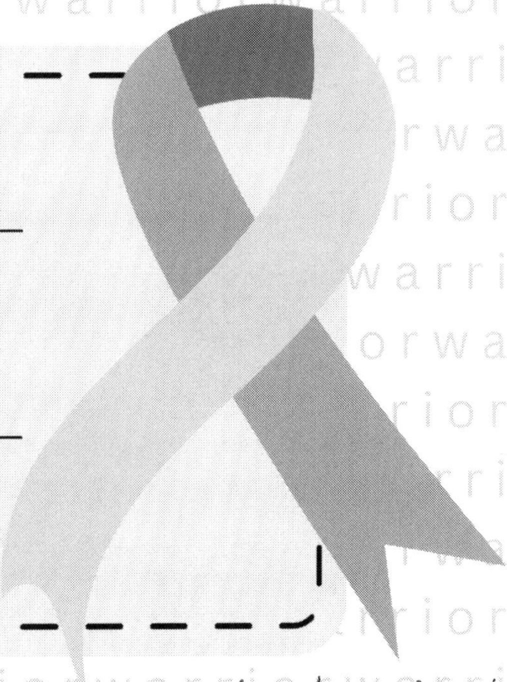

I wish I could take this diagnosis away from you. I'll be with you thru it all! Please use this book whenever you need extra strength. God is with you — He can & will give you comfort.

♡ me

Copyright © 2024 by Biblical Teachings -All rights reserved.

No part of this book may be reproduced in any form or by any electronic or mechanical means, including information storage and retrieval systems, without written permission from the author, except for the use of brief quotations in a book review.

Under no circumstances will any blame or legal responsibility be held against the publisher, or author, for any damages, reparation, or monetary loss due to the information contained within this book, either directly or indirectly.

Legal Notice:

This book is copyright protected. It is only for personal use. You cannot amend, distribute, sell, use, quote, or paraphrase any part, or the content within this book, without the author or publisher's permission.

Disclaimer Notice:

Please note that the information contained within this document is for educational and entertainment purposes only. All effort has been executed to present accurate, up-to-date, reliable, complete information. No warranties of any kind are declared or implied. Readers acknowledge that the author is not rendering legal, financial, medical, or professional advice. The content within this book has been derived from various sources. Please consult a licensed professional before attempting any techniques outlined in this book.

By reading this document, the reader agrees that under no circumstances is the author responsible for any losses, direct or indirect, that are incurred due to the use of the information in this document, including, but not limited to, errors, omissions, or inaccuracies.

CONTENTS

A Journey of Courage	ix
1. The Moment That Changed Everything	1
2. Telling Loved Ones	3
3. Confronting Worst-Case Scenarios	5
4. Understanding Your Diagnosis	7
5. Emily's Story - Finding Her Tribe	9
6. Why Me? Wrestling with Unfairness	11
7. God's Presence in the Chaos	13
8. One Step at a Time	15
9. Maria's Story - Holding Onto Light in the Darkness	17
10. The First Steps of Treatment	24
11. Trusting Your Medical Team	26
12. Samantha's Story - The First Day of Chemo	28
13. Finding Stability	31
14. Strength for the Journey	33
15. Accepting Help	35
16. God's Healing Touch	37
17. Jane's Story - Celebrating Small Wins	39
18. Finding Peace in Prayer	41
19. Coping with Physical Changes	48
20. Finding Strength When You're Exhausted	50
21. Linda's Story - Eating When It's Hard	52
22. Loving Yourself Through Changes	54
23. Pain Management	56
24. Naomi's Story - Staying Connected When You Feel Alone	58
25. Riding the Emotional Waves	61
26. Restless Nights	63
27. Financial Strain	65
28. More Than a Patient	67
Light the Path for Another Woman on her Cancer Journey	72
29. Halfway There	76

30. Trusting the Process	78
31. Brianna's Story - Dealing with Setbacks	80
32. Finding Energy to Keep Going	82
33. Hope on Hard Days	85
34. Allowing Yourself to Be Human	87
35. Divine Strength	89
36. Words to Lift Your Spirit	91
37. Olivia's Story - Strength in Numbers	93
38. Walking by Faith	95
39. Seeing the Light	102
40. Preparing for the Next Steps	104
41. Amelia's Story - Pushing Through the Last Stages	107
42. Faith in the Finish Line	110
43. God's Promises	112
44. Caroline's Story - Reflecting on the Journey	114
45. Joy in Small Moments	116
46. Building New Dreams	118
47. Seeking Guidance for the Next Phase	120
48. Adjusting to Life After Treatment	126
49. Dealing with Fear of Recurrence	128
50. Laura's Story - Continuing Self-Care	131
51. Recovering Mentally and Spiritually	133
52. A Future Beyond Cancer	135
53. Yasmin's Story - Managing Long-Term Side Effects	137
54. Rebuilding Relationships	140
55. Returning to the Workplace	142
56. Physical Rehabilitation	144
57. Celebrating Survivorship	147
Pass On the Blessings	152
And So, The Journey Continues...	155

BIBLE STUDY
-Starter Kit-

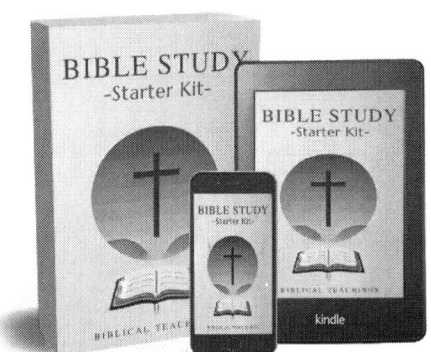

Discover a **<u>Simple</u>**, **<u>Powerful</u>** Way to Study
<u>The Bible</u>

- *No More Guesswork* - Learn to Explore the Bible **with Confidence** and Clarity.

- Discover a Study Method That *Fits Seamlessly into Your Busy Life* - **Without the Overwhelm**.

- **Build a Bible Study Routine** *You'll Actually Look Forward To* - Not Just Another Task on Your To-Do List.

<u>SCAN THE QR CODE</u> FOR YOUR <u>FREE</u> COPY

A JOURNEY OF COURAGE

Welcome to *'The Devotional for Women with Cancer.'* This book is here to walk alongside you during times that may feel overwhelming and uncertain. Whether you've just received a diagnosis, are undergoing treatment, or are navigating life after cancer, this devotional is crafted to be a source of gentle comfort and practical support tailored to your journey.

Inside these pages, you'll find devotions lovingly written to uplift you through the physical, emotional, and spiritual challenges of cancer. Each devotion is grounded in scripture and enriched with real stories, offering a heartfelt connection to your experiences.

We know that cancer can shake your world in ways you never imagined. It's not just about the physical struggles, emotions, and spiritual questions that arise. This devotional is here to be a safe space—a comforting companion where you can pause, reflect, and find moments of peace. We hope these devotions will help you feel God's loving presence and bring you hope and courage, no matter where you are on your journey.

How to Use This Book:

1. **Go at Your Own Pace:** This journey is uniquely yours, and there's no right or wrong way to use this book. Take your time, read a devotion when it feels right, and let it speak to your heart. This book is here whether you read daily, weekly, or whenever you need peace.
2. **Begin with Scripture:** Each devotion begins with a Bible verse chosen to offer comfort and strength. Let these words gently remind you of God's care and love for you.
3. **Engage with the Devotional Insight:** These insights are meant to resonate with your experiences, offering wisdom and encouragement. Let the stories and reflections be a gentle guide, helping you navigate the complexities of this journey.
4. **Reflect and Relate:** After each devotion, take a moment to reflect. The prompts are here to help you process your thoughts and feelings, offering a space to relate the insights to your journey.
5. **Prayer Time:** Conclude with a prayer, opening your heart to God's comforting presence. These prayers are simple, heartfelt words to help you feel supported and loved.
6. **Workbook Pages:** At the end of each section, you'll find a workbook page designed for you to reflect, journal, or take action based on what you've learned. Use these pages to apply the insights from the devotional and grow closer together as you deepen your connection with God.

You'll find themes of faith, resilience, and hope throughout these devotions. Whether it's dealing with the side effects of treatment, facing emotional ups and downs, or seeking peace amidst the chaos, these devotions are here to uplift you.

This journey requires immense strength and courage, and feeling scared or uncertain is okay. We pray that these devotions will provide gentle comfort and strength, helping you feel less alone and more connected to God's love. Remember, you are not alone. God's love is constant, and His presence is with you every step of the way.

Let's walk this path together, finding hope and healing during challenges. We're here with you every step of the way.

P.S. *All scripture quotations are taken from the Holy Bible, New International Version (NIV), unless otherwise noted.*

Diagnosis & Initial Shock

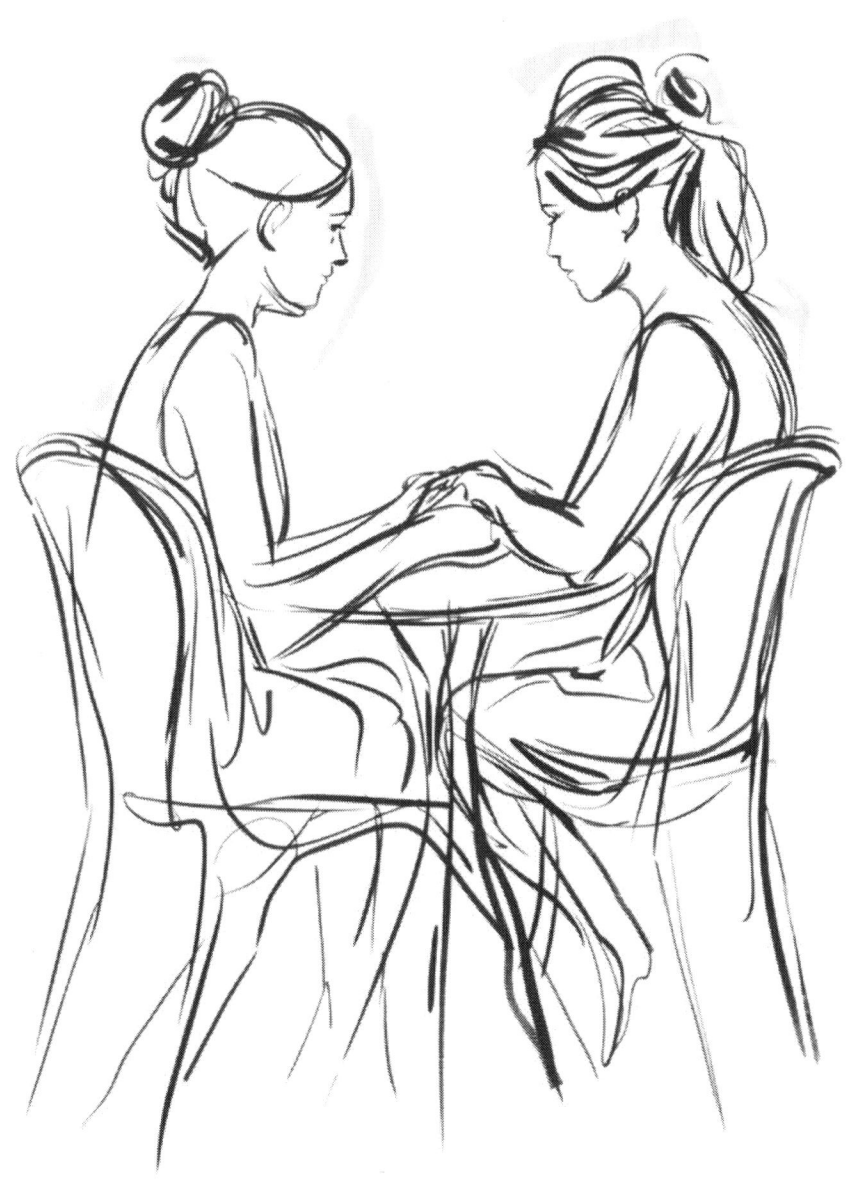

THE MOMENT THAT CHANGED EVERYTHING

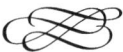

"The Lord is close to the brokenhearted and saves those who are crushed in spirit."

— PSALM 34:18

The doctor's words hung in the air, heavy and unrelenting. *"You have cancer."* In that instant, your world shifted, and a flood of emotions rushed in—fear, disbelief, anger, sorrow. Everything you had planned, every dream you held dear, seemed to crumble at your feet.

As you sit in the stillness, trying to process this life-altering news, it feels like you are navigating through a storm. Yet, in the midst of this storm, there is a profound truth that offers comfort: God is close to the brokenhearted. He sees your pain, understands your fears, and is right there with you in this moment of despair.

Take a deep breath and let this truth sink in. God's presence is not distant or indifferent; it is near and compassionate. He is there to save those who are crushed in spirit. This diagnosis does not define you, and it does not dictate the entirety of your story. God's love and comfort are your anchors, holding you steady as you face this new reality.

Remember, it's okay to feel broken, to grieve, and to be overwhelmed. Allow yourself to feel these emotions, but also allow God's presence to fill the cracks of your broken heart with His healing love.

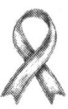

Prayer

Heavenly Father, I am overwhelmed and scared by the news I have received. My heart feels broken, and my spirit is crushed. But I hold onto Your promise that You are close to the brokenhearted. Please comfort me in this time of fear and uncertainty. Wrap me in Your love, and give me the strength to face each day. Help me to feel Your presence and to trust that You are with me every step of the way. Amen.

Reflection

- How do you feel God's presence in your life right now?

- What fears and emotions do you need to bring to Him for comfort and healing?

- *What do I want to remember about the way this moment redefined my relationship with God?*

_____

_____

_____

_____

_____

TELLING LOVED ONES

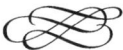

> *"Carry each other's burdens, and in this way you will fulfill the law of Christ."*
>
> — GALATIANS 6:2

The thought of telling your family and friends about your diagnosis feels almost as overwhelming as the diagnosis itself. You worry about their reactions, their pain, and how this news will affect them. But in this moment, remember that you don't have to carry this burden alone.

The Bible reminds us in Galatians 6:2 to carry each other's burdens. This isn't just a call to help others; it's also a reminder that it's okay to lean on those who love us. Sharing your burden with your loved ones can bring a profound sense of relief and support.

When you share your diagnosis, you might be surprised at the strength and comfort your loved ones can provide. They can become your pillars of support, offering prayers, helping with daily tasks, and simply being there to listen. Allow them to fulfill the law of Christ by carrying this burden with you.

It can help to find a quiet, comfortable place to talk. Start by being honest about your feelings and letting them know that you need their support. It's okay to show your vulnerability; your loved ones care for you and will want to help. You might also consider writing down what you want to say beforehand to organize your thoughts and ease the conversation.

You are not alone in this journey. Let the people who care about you in, let them help carry this load, and in doing so, you will find a community of support and love surrounding you.

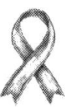

Prayer

Dear Lord, the thought of telling my loved ones about my diagnosis is overwhelming. Please give me the courage and the words to share this news with them. Help me to lean on those who love me and to allow them to support me through this journey. Thank You for placing people in my life who care for me deeply. Help me to feel their love and support, and remind me that we are carrying this burden together, with You guiding us. Amen.

Reflection

- Who do you need to tell about your diagnosis?

- How can you allow others to help carry your burden during this time?

_____

_____

_____

_____

CONFRONTING WORST-CASE SCENARIOS

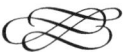

"Even though I walk through the darkest valley, I will fear no evil, for you are with me; your rod and your staff, they comfort me."

— PSALM 23:4

When I received my diagnosis, my mind immediately spiraled into the worst-case scenarios. *"What if the treatment doesn't work? What if the cancer spreads? What if I don't have much time left?"* These fears consumed me, making it hard to see beyond the shadows of my anxiety.

In those moments of darkness, I clung to Psalm 23:4. Walking through this valley, I realized I wasn't walking alone. God was with me, offering His comfort and strength. He didn't promise a life without valleys, but He did promise His presence in the midst of them.

To confront these fears, I started by acknowledging them. I allowed myself to feel the fear, but I didn't let it paralyze me. I prayed, asking God to replace my fear with His peace. I also sought out information about my condition and treatment options from reliable sources, which helped me feel more in control.

Talking to my doctors and asking questions gave me clarity and reduced my anxiety. They reassured me about the treatment process and outcomes. I also reached out to support groups, finding solace in the stories of others who had faced similar fears and come out stronger on the other side.

Remember, it's okay to have fears, but don't let them control you. Lean on God's promise that He is with you, even in the darkest valleys. His comfort and guidance will see you through.

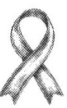

Prayer

Lord, my fears often overwhelm me, and I find myself imagining the worst-case scenarios. Help me to confront these fears with Your strength. Remind me that I am not alone in this journey, and that Your presence is my comfort. Replace my anxiety with Your peace, and help me to trust in Your plan for my life. Amen.

Reflection

- What are your biggest fears right now, and how can you bring them to God?

- How can seeking information and support help you confront these fears?

- *What do I want to remember about the courage I showed and the peace I found by facing my fears with faith and support?*

_____

_____

UNDERSTANDING YOUR DIAGNOSIS

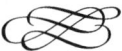

"For the Spirit God gave us does not make us timid, but gives us power, love, and self-discipline."

— 2 TIMOTHY 1:7

When you first hear your diagnosis, the medical jargon and flood of information can be overwhelming. It's easy to feel lost and powerless in the face of so much uncertainty. But remember, God has given you a spirit not of fear, but of power, love, and self-discipline.

Take a moment to breathe and center yourself. Start by asking your doctor to explain your diagnosis in simple terms. It can be helpful to bring a notebook or record the conversation to review later. Don't hesitate to ask for written materials or trusted online resources to better understand your condition.

Consider making a list of questions before your appointments. What does the diagnosis mean? What are the treatment options? What are the side effects? Having a prepared list can help ensure you get the information you need. Bringing a loved one to your appointments can also provide emotional support and help you remember the details discussed.

It's natural to feel anxious about the unknown, but educating yourself can empower you. Each bit of information you gather equips you to make informed decisions about your treatment. Take it one step at a time, and give yourself grace as you navigate this new terrain.

Rely on the spirit God has given you—a spirit of power, love, and self-discipline. This spirit will guide you, strengthen you, and help you face each day with confidence and peace.

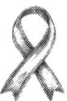

Prayer

Dear God, I feel overwhelmed by the information and uncertainty of my diagnosis. Help me to understand my condition and guide me in asking the right questions. Give me the strength and clarity to navigate this journey with confidence. Surround me with supportive people who can help me along the way. Amen.

Reflection

- What questions do you have about your diagnosis that you need answers to?

- How can you use the power, love, and self-discipline God has given you to seek understanding and clarity?

EMILY'S STORY - FINDING HER TRIBE

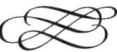

"Therefore encourage one another and build each other up, just as in fact you are doing."

— 1 THESSALONIANS 5:11

Emily felt utterly alone when she first received her diagnosis. The weight of the news was heavy, and even though she had family around her, she longed for someone who truly understood what she was going through. During a routine check-up, her nurse mentioned a local support group for women with cancer.

With some hesitation, Emily decided to attend a meeting. She walked into the room filled with women of various ages, all sharing the same burden. As they began to speak, Emily felt an overwhelming sense of connection and relief. These women spoke her language; they understood the fears, the uncertainties, and the hope that she held.

"At first, I wasn't sure if I could relate to anyone," Emily recalls. *"But as soon as they started sharing their stories, I realized they were going through the same things I was. It was like a weight lifted off my shoulders—finally, I wasn't alone."*

BIBLICAL TEACHINGS

Over time, this group became Emily's tribe. They prayed together, celebrated small victories, and provided shoulders to cry on during the tough days. They shared tips on managing side effects, recipes for nutritious meals, and words of encouragement that only someone walking the same path could offer.

"Finding this group changed everything for me," Emily says with a smile. *"I no longer felt isolated; instead, I was surrounded by a community that lifted me up and helped me face each day with renewed strength and courage. This tribe became my lifeline, showing me that I didn't have to walk this journey alone."*

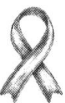

Prayer

Lord, thank You for the gift of community and support. Help me to find my tribe, a group of people who understand my journey and can offer me encouragement and strength. Guide me to those who will lift me up and walk alongside me through this challenge. Amen.

Reflection

- Who are the people in your life that you can turn to for support?

- How can you reach out and connect with others who are going through a similar experience?

_____

_____

_____

_____

WHY ME? WRESTLING WITH UNFAIRNESS

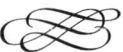

"The Lord is close to the brokenhearted and saves those who are crushed in spirit."

— PSALM 34:18

"Why me?" It's a question that has echoed in my mind since the day I was diagnosed. I've always tried to live a good life, to do what's right. So why did this happen to me? This sense of unfairness can be overwhelming, and it's hard not to feel singled out by this diagnosis.

In my struggle with this question, I've found comfort in Psalm 34:18. God doesn't promise us a life free from pain or hardship, but He does promise to be close to the brokenhearted. He sees our pain, our confusion, and our sense of injustice. He is there, offering comfort and understanding, even when we don't have all the answers.

I've learned to bring my honest feelings to God, to tell Him about my anger, my sadness, and my confusion. I've found that in these moments of raw honesty, His presence feels closest. It's in these times that I can sense His peace, even when I don't understand His plan.

BIBLICAL TEACHINGS

I also try to focus on the ways God's presence has been evident in my journey. The unexpected acts of kindness from strangers, the deepened relationships with friends and family, and the strength I've discovered within myself—all these are signs of God working in my life, even amidst the unfairness.

"Why me?" I may never fully understand the answer. But I do know that I am not alone. God is with me, close to my broken heart, and He is carrying me through this.

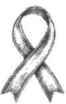

Prayer

Dear God, I struggle with the unfairness of this diagnosis and the question of why me. Help me to feel Your presence and to trust in Your plan, even when I don't understand. Comfort my broken heart and give me the strength to face each day with faith. Amen.

Reflection

• How can you bring your honest feelings to God and seek His comfort?

• In what ways have you seen God's presence in your life, even amidst the struggles?

_____

_____

_____

_____

_____

GOD'S PRESENCE IN THE CHAOS

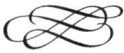

"Be still, and know that I am God."

— PSALM 46:10

In the midst of the chaos that a cancer diagnosis brings, it can be incredibly challenging to find a moment of peace. Appointments, treatments, phone calls, and the constant hum of worry can make you feel like you're caught in a storm. But even in the storm, God is with you. His presence is constant, unwavering, and He calls you to find stillness in Him.

Imagine for a moment that you are in the eye of a hurricane. The winds are raging around you, but right where you stand, there is calm. This is where God invites you to be—still and aware of His presence. Take a few moments each day to quiet your mind and heart. Find a place where you can sit quietly and breathe deeply, focusing on the truth that God is with you.

Even when everything feels out of control, remind yourself that God is your anchor. He is not distant or detached from your pain; He is right there with you, offering peace that surpasses understanding.

When you feel overwhelmed, speak the words of Psalm 46:10 to yourself: "Be still, and know that I am God." Let these words be a balm to your soul, grounding you in His love and care.

Lean into His presence in the small, quiet moments. It might be a silent prayer, a whispered plea for strength, or a moment of reflection on a scripture that brings you comfort. These moments are where you will find God's peace, even in the chaos.

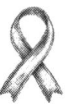

Prayer

Heavenly Father, in the midst of the chaos and uncertainty, help me to be still and recognize Your presence. Calm my anxious heart and fill me with Your peace. Remind me that You are with me, anchoring me with Your love and strength. Amen.

Reflection

- How can you create moments of stillness in your daily routine to feel God's presence?

- What scripture or prayer brings you comfort and helps you feel anchored in God's peace?

_____

_____

_____

_____

_____

_____

ONE STEP AT A TIME

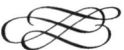

"Therefore do not worry about tomorrow, for tomorrow will worry about itself. Each day has enough trouble of its own."

— MATTHEW 6:34

It's easy to become overwhelmed by the enormity of what lies ahead. The treatment plans, the side effects, the what-ifs—they all pile up, creating a mountain of worry and fear. But God encourages you to take it one step at a time. Focus on today and trust that He will give you the strength you need for each moment.

Instead of letting your mind race ahead to all the possible outcomes, concentrate on the present. What do you need to do today? Maybe it's just getting through one appointment, one meal, or one conversation. Break your day into manageable parts, and tackle each task with the understanding that God is with you, providing what you need for that moment.

When you feel yourself starting to spiral into worry, take a deep breath and bring your thoughts back to the present. Remind yourself that God's grace is sufficient for today. Trust that He will take care of tomorrow and that His strength is enough to get you through this day.

Give yourself permission to take small steps and to rest when needed. Healing and coping with a cancer diagnosis is a journey that requires patience and self-compassion. Each small step forward, no matter how insignificant it may seem, is a victory. Trust that God is walking with you, guiding your steps, and holding you up with His unfailing love.

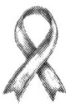

Prayer

Lord, help me to focus on today and not be overwhelmed by the worries of tomorrow. Give me the strength and grace I need for each moment. Remind me that You are with me every step of the way, providing for my needs and calming my fears. Amen.

Reflection

- How can you break down your day into manageable steps to reduce anxiety?

- What small victories can you celebrate today as you rely on God's grace?

- *What do I want to remember about the strength I've gained by simply taking one step at a time?*

_____

_____

_____

MARIA'S STORY - HOLDING ONTO LIGHT IN THE DARKNESS

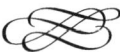

"The light shines in the darkness, and the darkness has not overcome it."

— JOHN 1:5

When Maria was diagnosed with cancer, the news felt like a heavy curtain of darkness descending upon her life. She struggled to find hope amidst the fear and uncertainty. But through her journey, Maria discovered that even the smallest glimmer of light could pierce through the darkest times.

Maria began to notice the little things that brought light into her life—a kind word from a friend, a sunny day, a moment of laughter. She started keeping a journal to write down these moments of light, however small they seemed. This practice helped her to shift her focus from the overwhelming darkness to the small, but significant, sources of hope and joy.

She also leaned heavily on her faith. The verse from John 1:5 became her mantra: *"The light shines in the darkness, and the darkness has not overcome it."* Maria reminded herself daily that no matter how dark things seemed, the light of God's love and hope was stronger and would not be extinguished.

Maria's church community rallied around her, offering prayers, meals, and companionship. Their support was a tangible reminder of God's light shining through others. Even on her hardest days, Maria clung to the light, knowing that the darkness could not overcome it.

Through her journey, Maria learned that hope is not the absence of darkness, but the presence of light that the darkness cannot conquer. Her story is a testament to the power of holding onto hope, even when everything seems bleak.

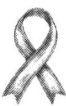

Prayer

Dear Lord, when the darkness of fear and uncertainty feels overwhelming, help me to see the light of Your love and hope. Remind me that Your light shines brightly, even in the darkest times, and that the darkness will not overcome it. Surround me with Your presence and the support of others, and help me to cling to the hope that You provide. Amen.

Reflection

- What small moments of light and hope can you find in your daily life?
- How can you focus on these moments to help you through the darker times?

_____

_____

_____

DATE

S M T W T F S

Finding Light in the Darkness

NOTICE JOY

Pause during your day to appreciate something that brings you joy, hope, or peace. Describe the moment in one sentence:

_____
_____
_____

GRATITUDE JAR

Find a small jar or container. Each day, write down something you're thankful for on a small piece of paper and place it in the jar.

How does it feel to express gratitude this way?

_____
_____
_____
_____

CONNECT WITH NATURE

Spend a few moments outside, noticing the beauty of the natural world around you—a flower, the sky, or the sound of birds.

How does being in nature affect your mood?

_____
_____
_____

DRAW THE LIGHT

Imagine a small light inside you, growing brighter and filling you with warmth and peace. Now, draw what this light looks like to you. <u>Use any colors or shapes that come to mind.</u>

How do you feel after drawing it?

_____
_____
_____
_____
_____

*Even in dark times, God's love shines.
Keep noticing and appreciating those
little moments of light."*

Starting Treatment

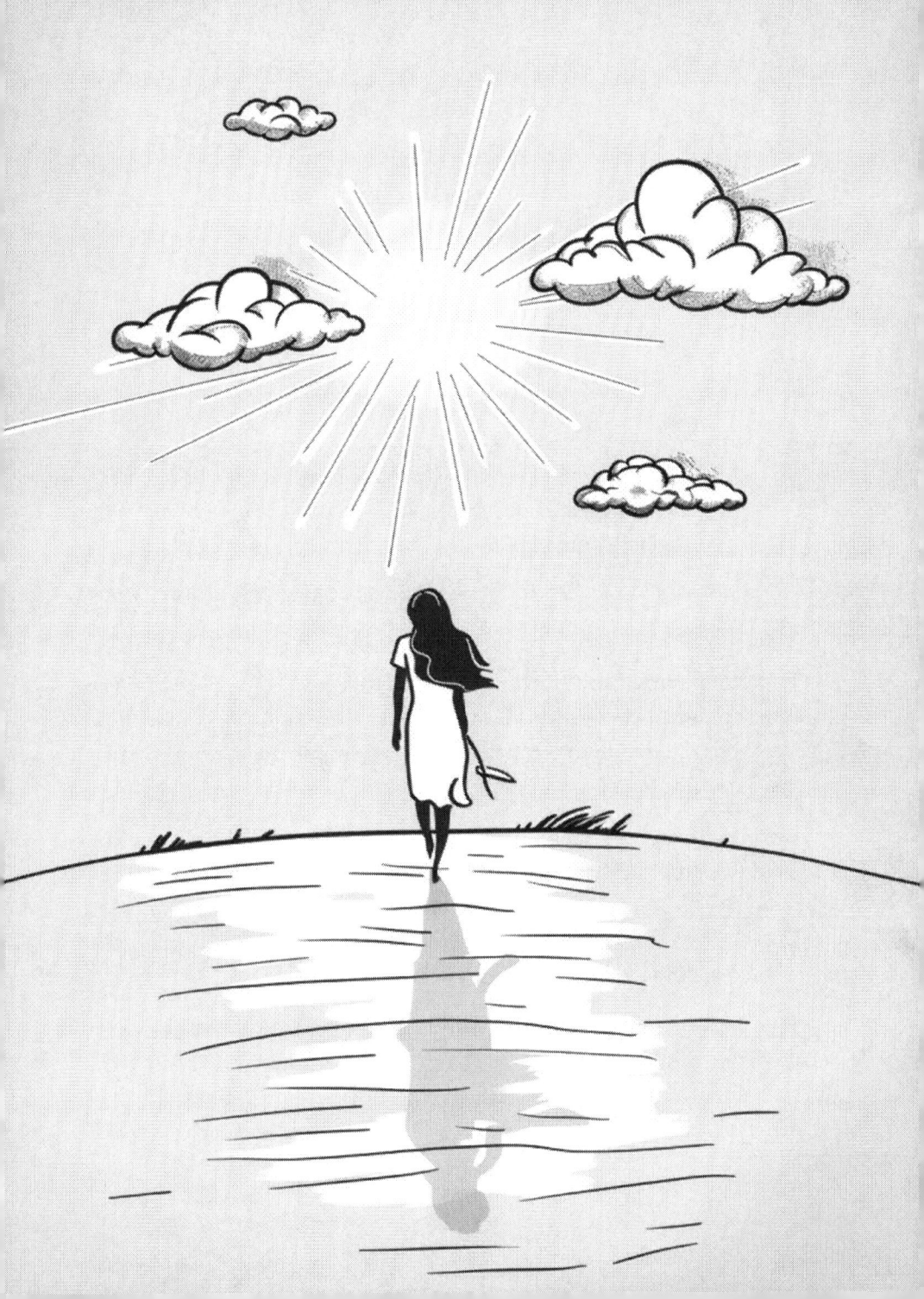

THE FIRST STEPS OF TREATMENT

> *"The Lord himself goes before you and will be with you; he will never leave you nor forsake you. Do not be afraid; do not be discouraged."*
>
> — DEUTERONOMY 31:8

The day I started my treatment was filled with a mix of emotions. Fear, anxiety, hope—they all swirled together as I took those first steps into the treatment center. It felt like stepping into the unknown, and I couldn't help but wonder what lay ahead.

During those moments of uncertainty, I found solace in Deuteronomy 31:8. The assurance that God goes before me and remains with me provided immense comfort. Knowing that He would never abandon me gave me the courage to move forward, even when fear threatened to hold me back.

The first steps were the hardest. I felt overwhelmed by the medical terms, the machinery, and the unfamiliar faces. But as I sat in the treatment chair, I began to notice the kindness in the eyes of the nurses and the reassuring words of the doctors.

Each interaction reminded me that I was not alone in this journey.

I learned to take it one day at a time, trusting that God was guiding my steps. Each day brought new challenges, but also new strength and resilience. I found that by leaning on God's promise, I could face each step with a bit more courage and hope.

Starting treatment is daunting, but remember that God is with you in every moment. He goes before you, preparing the way, and He will walk with you through every step of this journey.

Prayer

Heavenly Father, as I begin my treatment, help me to trust that You are with me every step of the way. Give me the strength and courage to face each day, and remind me that I am not alone. Thank You for Your promise to never leave me nor forsake me. Amen.

Reflection

- What fears do you have about starting treatment, and how can you bring them to God?
- How can you remind yourself of God's presence and promises as you take these first steps?

_____

_____

_____

_____

_____

TRUSTING YOUR MEDICAL TEAM

"Plans fail for lack of counsel, but with many advisers they succeed."

— PROVERBS 15:22

As you navigate your treatment journey, it's crucial to trust the medical team that is dedicated to your care. These professionals have spent years training and are equipped with the knowledge and skills to guide you through this challenging time. It's natural to feel anxious about the process, but remember that you are in capable hands.

Start by building a relationship with your doctors and nurses. Ask questions and seek clarity about your treatment plan. Understanding the steps and the reasons behind them can provide a sense of control and trust. Don't hesitate to ask for explanations in simpler terms if medical jargon becomes overwhelming.

Your medical team is there to support you, not just through treatment, but emotionally as well. Share your concerns and fears with them; they can offer reassurances and adjust your care to better suit your needs. Remember, they are part of your support system, working tirelessly to help you fight this battle.

Proverbs 15:22 reminds us of the importance of counsel and advisers. Your medical team is your counsel in this journey. Trust their expertise and lean on their guidance. This trust will help you feel more secure and less alone in your fight against cancer.

Prayer

Lord, help me to trust the medical team You have placed in my life. Give me the courage to ask questions and seek understanding. Help me to feel secure in their care and to trust that they are working for my good. Thank You for providing knowledgeable and compassionate people to support me through this journey. Amen.

Reflection

- How can you build trust with your medical team and feel more secure in their care?

- What questions or concerns do you have that you can bring to your medical team for clarity and reassurance?

_____

_____

_____

_____

_____

SAMANTHA'S STORY - THE FIRST DAY OF CHEMO

"When you pass through the waters, I will be with you; and when you pass through the rivers, they will not sweep over you."

— ISAIAH 43:2

Samantha walked into the chemotherapy clinic with her heart pounding in her chest. The sterile smell, the beeping machines, and the sight of other patients hooked up to IVs filled her with dread. This was her first day of chemo, and she felt a wave of fear wash over her.

As she settled into the chair, a nurse with a kind smile approached her. The nurse explained each step of the process, what the medications were for, and what side effects she might experience. Samantha felt a bit of her anxiety lift as the nurse spoke calmly and clearly. She appreciated the transparency and the effort to make her comfortable.

"I was terrified walking in," Samantha recalls. "But when the nurse started explaining everything, I felt some of that fear start to fade. Just knowing what to expect helped me feel a little more in control."

During the infusion, Samantha brought along a cozy blanket, a book, and some music to help pass the time. She noticed other patients doing similar things—some were knitting, others were watching movies, and a few were chatting with companions. It was a small comfort to see that she wasn't alone in this experience.

"Seeing others there, going through the same thing, made me realize that I wasn't alone," she says. *"We were all facing this together, and that brought me some peace."*

Throughout the day, Samantha kept Isaiah 43:2 in her mind. The verse reminded her that God was with her, even in this intimidating setting. As the medication flowed into her veins, she visualized God's presence surrounding her, giving her strength and peace.

By the end of the day, Samantha was tired but felt a sense of accomplishment. *"I did it,"* she reflects. *"I faced my fear and made it through my first chemo session. I know the road ahead is long, but I can take it one step at a time, with God's promise of presence and support guiding me."*

Prayer

Dear God, the first day of chemotherapy is daunting and filled with fear. Please be with me, giving me strength and peace. Help me to find comfort in Your presence and in the care of those around me. Thank You for walking with me through this challenging time. Amen.

Reflection

- What are your fears about starting chemotherapy, and how can you bring them to God?

- How can you prepare yourself, both physically and mentally, for your first treatment session?

BIBLICAL TEACHINGS

• What do I want to remember about the courage I had as I faced my fears and took the first step in my treatment journey?

FINDING STABILITY

"Commit your work to the Lord, and your plans will be established."

— PROVERBS 16:3

As you begin your treatment journey, finding stability can feel like trying to balance on a moving ship. The routines you once knew may no longer fit, and it's easy to feel unmoored. But creating a new routine can bring a sense of control and peace amidst the uncertainty.

Start by setting small, manageable goals each day. These could be as simple as waking up at the same time, taking a short walk, or spending a few moments in prayer. Establishing these small rituals can help anchor your day and provide a sense of normalcy.

Don't be afraid to adjust your routines as needed. Listen to your body and give yourself grace on the days when things don't go as planned. It's okay to rest and to ask for help when you need it.

Include time for things that bring you joy and relaxation. Whether it's reading a book, listening to music, or spending time with loved ones, these moments of happiness can be powerful sources of strength.

Commit your new routines to the Lord. Pray for guidance and strength to maintain them, and trust that God will help establish your plans. With His help, you can find stability and peace, even in the midst of treatment.

Prayer

Lord, help me to find stability in my daily routines as I undergo treatment. Guide me in creating a new rhythm that brings peace and strength. Give me the grace to adjust as needed and the wisdom to include moments of joy and relaxation. I commit my plans to You, trusting that You will establish them. Amen.

Reflection

- What small routines can you establish to bring stability to your day?

- How can you invite God into your daily plans and seek His guidance?

_____

_____

_____

_____

STRENGTH FOR THE JOURNEY

"I can do all this through him who gives me strength."

— PHILIPPIANS 4:13

When I first heard the words, *"You have cancer,"* I felt an overwhelming wave of fear and uncertainty. But as I embarked on this journey, I discovered a strength within me that I never knew existed. It wasn't a strength I found on my own, but one that came from God.

Philippians 4:13 became my lifeline. I repeated it to myself in the quiet moments before treatments, during the long nights, and on days when I felt too weak to move. *"I can do all this through him who gives me strength."* These words reminded me that I was not relying on my own strength, but on God's boundless power and love.

Resilience isn't about being unbreakable; it's about trusting God to put the pieces back together when you feel shattered. It's about facing each day with the knowledge that God is with you, providing the strength you need to keep going.

There were days when I felt like giving up, but in those moments, I turned to prayer and scripture. I found encouragement in the stories of others who had walked this path and emerged stronger. Their testimonies fueled my hope and reminded me that resilience is a journey of faith.

With each step, I learned to lean more on God and less on my own understanding. His strength carried me through the darkest valleys and helped me to see the light of hope ahead. Trusting in His strength allowed me to face each day with courage and determination.

Prayer

Heavenly Father, thank You for the strength You provide. Help me to rely on Your power and love as I navigate this journey. Give me the resilience to face each day with courage, and remind me that I can do all things through You. Strengthen my faith and fill me with Your peace. Amen.

Reflection

- How can you rely on God's strength in your daily challenges?
- What scriptures or prayers encourage you to build resilience?

_____

_____

_____

_____

_____

ACCEPTING HELP

"Bear one another's burdens, and so fulfill the law of Christ."

— GALATIANS 6:2

Accepting help can be one of the hardest things to do, especially when you're used to being independent. But in this season, leaning on your loved ones is not a sign of weakness—it's an act of strength and trust.

God designed us to live in community, to support one another through life's challenges. When you allow others to help you, you're giving them the opportunity to show Christ's love in action. It's a beautiful, reciprocal relationship where both the giver and receiver are blessed.

Start by being honest about your needs. Whether it's help with household chores, transportation to appointments, or simply having someone to talk to, let your loved ones know how they can support you. Remember, they care about you and want to help, but they might not know how unless you tell them.

It can be helpful to make a list of tasks you need assistance with. This can make it easier to delegate and ensure that you get the support you need. Don't hesitate to accept offers of help, and thank those who step in with gratitude and grace.

Galatians 6:2 encourages us to bear one another's burdens. By accepting help, you're allowing your loved ones to fulfill this biblical principle. Trust that God has placed these people in your life for a reason and let their support strengthen and uplift you.

Prayer

Lord, help me to accept the help of my loved ones with grace and gratitude. Give me the courage to ask for support when I need it and the humility to receive it. Thank You for surrounding me with people who care for me. Help me to lean on them and to feel Your love through their actions. Amen.

Reflection

- In what areas of your life do you need support, and how can you communicate this to your loved ones?

- How can accepting help deepen your relationships and bring you closer to those who care for you?

_____

_____

_____

_____

_____

GOD'S HEALING TOUCH

"He heals the brokenhearted and binds up their wounds."

— PSALM 147:3

When I was first diagnosed with cancer, I felt like my body had betrayed me. The treatments, the side effects, the constant doctor's visits—it all felt overwhelming. But through it all, I experienced God's healing touch in ways I never expected.

Psalm 147:3 became a source of comfort for me. It reminded me that God is a healer, not just of physical ailments, but of the broken heart and spirit. I started to see His healing in the small, everyday miracles. A day with less pain, a good report from the doctor, a moment of laughter with my family—each of these was a touch of God's healing in my life.

There were times when I felt utterly broken, but in those moments, I would feel a sense of peace and comfort that could only come from God. I realized that healing is not always about the absence of illness, but about the presence of God's love and care in the midst of it.

Prayer became my lifeline. I would sit quietly, placing my fears and pain into God's hands, and I could feel His presence surrounding me. Each prayer was like a balm to my wounded spirit, bringing me closer to the One who heals all wounds.

I learned to trust in God's timing and His ways. His healing might not always look like what we expect, but it is always perfect. He knows our needs better than we do, and His touch brings wholeness in the most profound ways.

Prayer

Heavenly Father, thank You for Your healing touch. Help me to trust in Your ways and Your timing. Heal my broken heart and spirit, and bring comfort and peace to my life. Remind me that You are always with me, binding up my wounds with Your love. Amen.

Reflection

- In what ways have you experienced God's healing touch in your life?

- How can you trust God's timing and His ways in your journey to healing?

_____

_____

_____

_____

_____

JANE'S STORY - CELEBRATING SMALL WINS

"Rejoice in the Lord always. I will say it again: Rejoice!"

— PHILIPPIANS 4:4

Jane had always been a strong and independent woman, but her cancer diagnosis had shaken her to the core. As she began her treatment journey, she found herself focusing on the daunting road ahead, often feeling overwhelmed by the enormity of it all. But then something changed.

One day, after a particularly tough treatment session, Jane's granddaughter brought her a drawing with the words *"You are my hero"* written in bright, cheerful colors. Jane felt a warmth spread through her heart.

"I realized that amidst the struggle, there were moments worth celebrating —small wins that brought joy and hope," Jane recalls.

She started to make it a habit to celebrate these small victories. *"I'd rejoice when I had the energy to take a short walk, when my appetite returned for my favorite meal, or when I enjoyed a pain-free day,"* she says.

"Each of these moments, no matter how small, became a beacon of hope and a reason to rejoice."

Her support group became a huge part of this new mindset. They shared their small wins at each meeting, lifting each other up and finding joy in each other's victories. This practice not only brought them closer but also filled their journey with positivity and gratitude.

Philippians 4:4 encouraged Jane to rejoice always, and she found that focusing on the small wins helped her do just that. *"It didn't mean that the journey was easy,"* Jane reflects, *"but it meant that joy was always present, ready to be embraced in the midst of it all."*

Prayer

Lord, help me to find joy in the small wins each day. Teach me to celebrate the little victories and to rejoice in Your goodness. Thank You for the moments of happiness and hope that remind me of Your presence. Fill my heart with gratitude and joy, even in the midst of challenges. Amen.

Reflection

- What small wins can you celebrate today?

- How can focusing on these victories bring more joy and positivity into your life?

_____

_____

_____

_____

FINDING PEACE IN PRAYER

"Do not be anxious about anything, but in every situation, by prayer and petition, with thanksgiving, present your requests to God."

— PHILIPPIANS 4:6

In the midst of treatment, anxiety can often feel overwhelming. The uncertainty, the physical toll, and the emotional rollercoaster can all weigh heavily on your heart. But God offers a powerful antidote to anxiety: prayer.

When you feel anxiety creeping in, take a moment to pause and turn to God in prayer. You don't need to have the perfect words; just speak from your heart. Tell Him about your fears, your worries, and your needs. God is always ready to listen and to provide His peace.

Philippians 4:6 reminds us to present our requests to God with thanksgiving. As you pray, also take time to thank Him for His faithfulness and the blessings you've experienced, no matter how small they may seem. Gratitude can shift your focus from what's causing anxiety to what is good and uplifting in your life.

Make prayer a regular part of your day. Find a quiet place where you can connect with God without distractions. Whether it's first thing in the morning, during a break in your day, or before you go to bed, these moments of prayer can become a sanctuary of peace.

Remember, prayer is not just about asking for help; it's also about finding solace in God's presence. As you pour out your heart to Him, let His peace wash over you, calming your fears and reassuring you of His love and care.

Prayer

Dear God, I come to You with my fears and anxieties, asking for Your peace to fill my heart. Help me to trust in Your care and to feel Your presence in every moment. Thank You for the blessings in my life and for listening to my prayers. May Your peace, which surpasses all understanding, guard my heart and mind. Amen.

Reflection

- How can you incorporate regular prayer into your daily routine to find peace?

- What are you thankful for today that you can include in your prayers?

- *What do I want to remember about the peace and comfort I've experienced through prayer during difficult times?*

_____

_____

_____

DATE

S M T W T F S

Finding Strength and Stability

SAY THANK YOU

Thank someone who has helped you.
Who did you thank? How did they respond?

Who I thanked:

_____
_____

Their response:

_____
_____
_____

MINDFUL BREATHING

Practice mindful breathing for a few minutes. Focus on your breath as it flows in and out, bringing calm and stability to your mind and body.

How did this practice help you feel more centered?

_____
_____
_____
_____
_____
_____
_____
_____

BUILD A COMFORT BOX

Create a small box filled with items that bring you comfort—like a favorite book, a candle, or photos of loved ones.

What items did you choose, and why?

Item	Why

Even during tough times, God's love brings peace. Find small moments of calm and gratitude to help you through.

Facing Challenges Head-On

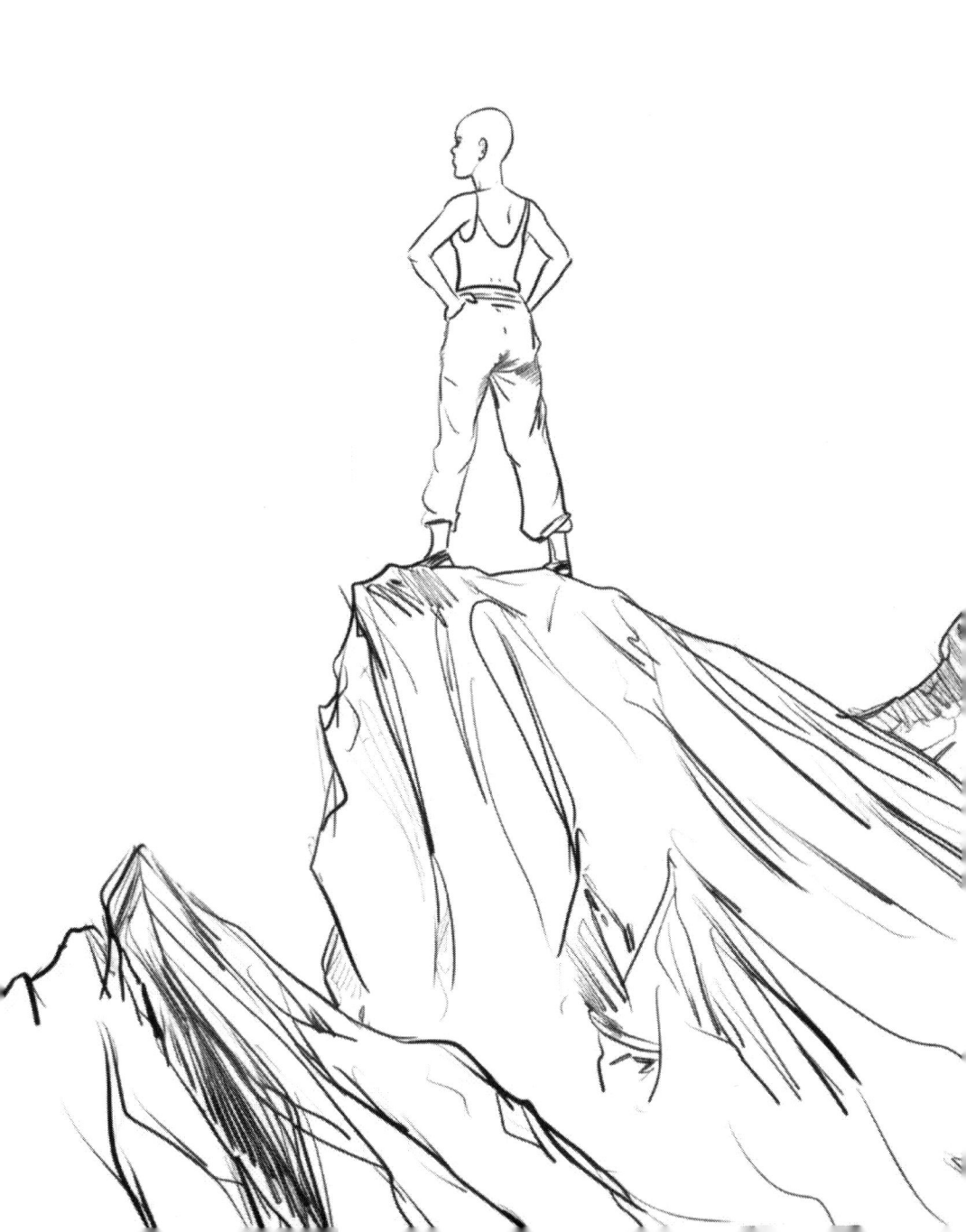

COPING WITH PHYSICAL CHANGES

"You are altogether beautiful, my darling; there is no flaw in you."

— SONG OF SOLOMON 4:7

The mirror became my enemy after my diagnosis - I barely recognized the person staring back at me. Each day, I watched as the treatments took their toll on my body. My hair, once thick and flowing, began to thin and fall out in clumps. My skin grew pale and dry, and the weight fluctuations left me feeling like a stranger in my own skin. The physical changes were a constant reminder of my battle with cancer, and they took a heavy toll on my self-esteem.

One morning, as I stared at my reflection with tears in my eyes, I remembered a verse from the Song of Solomon. *"You are altogether beautiful, my darling; there is no flaw in you."* It felt almost impossible to believe those words applied to me. How could I see myself as beautiful when cancer was stripping away so much of what I once was?

These words spoke directly to my heart. I realized that my worth and beauty were not tied to my hair or my physical appearance. God saw me as beautiful, even when I struggled to see it myself.

I decided to embrace this new look as part of my journey. I bought a few scarves and hats that made me feel stylish and comfortable. I even experimented with bold earrings and makeup, finding new ways to express my personality. Some days, I chose to go without any covering at all, proudly showing my strength and courage.

It wasn't easy, and there were still moments of sadness and frustration. But I learned to see my hair loss as a symbol of my fight, my resilience, and my faith. Every time I looked in the mirror, I reminded myself that God saw me as beautiful, and that gave me the confidence to see myself that way too.

Embracing a new look is a journey of acceptance and self-love. Trust that God sees you as flawless and beautiful, and let that truth guide you as you navigate this change.

Prayer

Dear Lord, help me to see myself through Your eyes. Remind me that my worth and beauty come from You, not from my outward appearance. Give me the strength to embrace this new look and to find confidence in Your love and affirmation. Amen.

Reflection

- How can you remind yourself of your worth and beauty in God's eyes?

- What steps can you take to embrace your new look and express your personality?

FINDING STRENGTH WHEN YOU'RE EXHAUSTED

"Come to me, all you who are weary and burdened, and I will give you rest."

— MATTHEW 11:28

The fatigue from treatment can be overwhelming. There are days when even getting out of bed feels like an insurmountable challenge. Your body is tired, your spirit is weary, and it's easy to feel like you have nothing left to give.

In these moments, remember the invitation Jesus extends in Matthew 11:28. He calls you to come to Him when you are weary and burdened, promising to give you rest. This rest isn't just physical; it's a deep, soul-refreshing rest that only God can provide.

Start by giving yourself permission to rest. It's okay to take a break, to slow down, and to prioritize your well-being. Listen to your body and respect its need for rest and recovery. Sometimes, the most powerful thing you can do is to allow yourself to rest in God's presence.

Find small ways to recharge. This might be taking a few minutes to breathe deeply and pray, listening to a favorite song, or simply sitting quietly in nature. These moments can provide a surprising amount of strength and refreshment.

Lean on the support of others. Let your loved ones help you with daily tasks and responsibilities. Accepting help is not a sign of weakness; it's a recognition that we all need support from time to time.

God's strength is made perfect in our weakness. When you feel you have no strength left, turn to Him. Allow His rest to rejuvenate you and His strength to carry you through.

Prayer

Lord, I am weary and exhausted. Please give me the rest and strength that I need. Help me to trust in Your promise and to lean on You when I feel burdened. Refresh my spirit and give me the courage to face each day with Your strength. Amen.

Reflection

- How can you incorporate moments of rest and rejuvenation into your day?

- In what ways can you lean on God and others for strength when you are feeling exhausted?

- *What do I want to remember about the strength I've found in God and through others when I've felt most drained?*

LINDA'S STORY - EATING WHEN IT'S HARD

◈

"So whether you eat or drink or whatever you do, do it all for the glory of God."

— 1 CORINTHIANS 10:31

Linda never thought something as simple as eating could become such a challenge. Chemotherapy had stolen her appetite and left her with a constant sense of nausea. Foods she once loved now turned her stomach, and mealtimes became a dreaded part of her day.

One afternoon, Linda's friend Sarah visited, bringing along homemade soup. Sarah had been through her own cancer journey and understood the struggle. She encouraged Linda to take small sips, reassuring her that it was okay to eat little by little. She shared her own experience of finding nourishment in small, manageable amounts and discovering what foods her body could tolerate.

Sarah reminded Linda of 1 Corinthians 10:31, encouraging her to see even this difficult part of her journey as an opportunity to honor God. *"Take it one bite at a time,"* Sarah said. *"God knows your struggle, and He's with you in this."*

Linda began to approach eating differently. She experimented with different foods, finding a few that she could enjoy without feeling sick. She learned to eat small, frequent meals instead of forcing herself to finish large portions. Each meal became an act of perseverance and faith, a way to care for her body and honor God, even in the midst of suffering.

She also prayed over her meals, asking God to bless the food and give her the strength to eat. Slowly, mealtime became less about the struggle and more about the small victories. Linda found that with God's help and the support of friends like Sarah, she could navigate this challenge one bite at a time.

Prayer

Dear God, eating has become a difficult part of my journey. Please help me find the strength to nourish my body, even when it's hard. Bless the food I eat and use it to give me the energy and health I need. Thank You for being with me in every struggle and for the support of friends who understand. Amen.

Reflection

- What small steps can you take to make eating more manageable and less stressful?

- How can you see even the act of eating as an opportunity to honor God in your journey?

_____

_____

_____

LOVING YOURSELF THROUGH CHANGES

⚜

"I praise you because I am fearfully and wonderfully made; your works are wonderful, I know that full well."

— PSALM 139:14

As you go through treatment, your body may change in ways you never expected. You might see scars, weight fluctuations, or other physical alterations that can be hard to accept. But remember, you are fearfully and wonderfully made, and God's works are wonderful—including you.

Start by giving yourself grace. Your body is fighting a tough battle, and every change is a testament to your strength and resilience. It's important to be kind to yourself and to recognize that beauty is not confined to physical appearance.

Take time each day to appreciate what your body is doing to heal. Look in the mirror and find one thing you can be grateful for. It might be the strength in your legs that carries you, the hands that hold your loved ones, or the eyes that see the world's beauty. Celebrate these aspects and thank God for them.

It's also helpful to surround yourself with positive influences. This might mean avoiding media that makes you feel bad about your body and instead filling your life with encouraging and affirming messages. Connect with friends who uplift you and remind you of your worth beyond physical appearance.

Loving yourself through these changes is a journey. Trust that God sees you as His beautiful creation, fearfully and wonderfully made. Embrace this truth and let it guide you as you navigate the physical changes brought on by treatment.

Prayer

Lord, help me to see myself through Your eyes. Remind me that I am fearfully and wonderfully made. Give me the grace to love myself through these changes and to find beauty in the strength and resilience You have given me. Thank You for my body and all it does to carry me through this journey. Amen.

Reflection

- What aspects of your body can you appreciate and thank God for today?

- How can you remind yourself of your worth beyond physical appearance?

_____

_____

_____

_____

PAIN MANAGEMENT

"He will wipe every tear from their eyes. There will be no more death or mourning or crying or pain, for the old order of things has passed away."

— REVELATION 21:4

Managing pain can be one of the most challenging aspects of your treatment journey. It can affect every part of your day, making even simple tasks feel overwhelming. But in these moments of discomfort, know that God is with you, offering comfort and hope.

Start by being proactive about your pain management. Talk openly with your medical team about what you're experiencing. They can help you find the right medications and strategies to manage your pain effectively. Don't hesitate to ask for adjustments if something isn't working—your comfort is important.

In addition to medical treatments, explore other methods that can bring relief. Gentle exercises, warm baths, meditation, and prayer can all be powerful tools in managing pain. Find what works for you and make it a part of your routine.

Remember Revelation 21:4, which promises a future without pain and suffering. While this promise refers to the eternal future, it can bring comfort in the present. God sees your pain and holds you through it. He offers a glimpse of His ultimate plan where there is no more suffering.

Lean into God's presence in moments of pain. Pray for His comfort and healing. Trust that He is with you, wiping away your tears and giving you strength to endure. Your pain is temporary, but God's love and comfort are eternal.

Prayer

Heavenly Father, please bring comfort to me in my pain. Help me to find effective ways to manage my discomfort and to lean on You for strength. Thank You for the promise of a future without pain and for Your presence with me now. Wrap me in Your love and help me to feel Your comforting touch. Amen.

Reflection

- What pain management strategies can you discuss with your medical team to improve your comfort?

- How can you incorporate prayer and other comforting practices into your daily routine to help manage pain?

_____

_____

_____

_____

NAOMI'S STORY - STAYING CONNECTED WHEN YOU FEEL ALONE

"And let us consider how we may spur one another on toward love and good deeds, not giving up meeting together, as some are in the habit of doing, but encouraging one another."

— HEBREWS 10:24-25

When Naomi was diagnosed with cancer, she felt an overwhelming sense of isolation. The physical toll of the illness and the treatment often left her feeling too exhausted to socialize. Friends seemed to drift away, not knowing how to offer support, and she found herself feeling alone in her struggle.

One day, Naomi's friend Jessica reached out. *"Naomi, I found this online support group for women with cancer. They've been through what you're going through. It might be really helpful,"* Jessica suggested. At first, Naomi was hesitant. She wasn't sure if she wanted to share her experiences with strangers. But with Jessica's encouragement, she decided to give it a try.

To her surprise, Naomi found the group to be incredibly supportive. These were people who truly understood what she was going through. In one of the first meetings, a woman shared, *"I know how hard it is to feel like no one understands. But here, we do."* They shared their stories, offered advice, and provided a space where she could express her fears and hopes without judgment. Through these virtual meetings, Naomi found a sense of community that she had been missing.

Inspired by Hebrews 10:24-25, Naomi realized the importance of staying connected. She began reaching out to friends and family more often, even if just for a short chat. She also discovered that small acts of connection—sending a text, writing a letter, or even a quick video call—could make a big difference in combating the feelings of isolation.

Naomi's journey taught her that staying connected, even in small ways, can bring immense encouragement and support. The love and good deeds shared within her community reminded her that she was not alone, and that together, they could spur each other on through love and encouragement.

Prayer

Dear Lord, help me to stay connected with those around me, even when I feel isolated. Guide me to the right support groups and communities where I can find encouragement and understanding. Thank You for the people You have placed in my life to support me on this journey. Amen.

Reflection

- Who can you reach out to today for support and connection?

BIBLICAL TEACHINGS

- How can small acts of connection help you feel less isolated and more supported?

• What do I want to remember about the courage it took to seek connection and the comfort I found in opening up to others?

RIDING THE EMOTIONAL WAVES

"The Lord is my strength and my shield; my heart trusts in him, and he helps me. My heart leaps for joy, and with my song I praise him."

— PSALM 28:7

Cancer treatment brought with it a tidal wave of emotions. Some days, I felt like I was riding a rollercoaster, with extreme highs and devastating lows. One moment, I would be filled with hope and determination, and the next, I would be overwhelmed with sadness and fear.

In those moments of emotional turmoil, I clung to Psalm 28:7. The Lord is my strength and my shield. These words reminded me that it was okay to feel these emotions, but I didn't have to face them alone. God was my constant, my anchor in the storm, providing strength and protection.

I learned to lean into my faith during these emotional waves. When I felt joy, I praised God for the good moments. When I felt sorrow, I poured out my heart to Him, knowing that He understood my pain. I also sought support from my loved ones, sharing my feelings and letting them pray for me and with me.

Journaling became a helpful tool as well. Writing down my thoughts and prayers allowed me to process my emotions and see God's faithfulness in every part of my journey. Even on the hardest days, I could look back and see how God had been my strength and shield.

Riding the emotional waves of cancer treatment is challenging, but remember that God is with you in every moment. Trust in Him, lean on Him, and let Him be your strength.

Prayer

Lord, my emotions feel overwhelming at times. Thank You for being my strength and shield. Help me to trust in You and to find comfort in Your presence. Guide me through the highs and lows, and fill my heart with Your peace. Amen.

Reflection

- How can you lean on God during your emotional highs and lows?

- What practices, like journaling or talking to loved ones, can help you process your emotions?

_____

_____

_____

_____

RESTLESS NIGHTS

"In peace I will lie down and sleep, for you alone, Lord, make me dwell in safety."

— PSALM 4:8

Restless nights are a common companion during cancer treatment. Anxiety, discomfort, and a racing mind can make it hard to find the rest you so desperately need. But even in these sleepless hours, God offers His peace and comfort.

When you find yourself tossing and turning, try to create a calming bedtime routine. This might include gentle stretches, a warm bath, or listening to soothing music. Find what helps you unwind and make it a nightly ritual.

Turn to prayer and scripture during these moments of restlessness. Psalm 4:8 is a powerful reminder that you can lie down in peace because the Lord makes you dwell in safety. Meditate on these words, letting them fill your heart and mind with God's promise of protection and peace.

Sometimes, it helps to keep a journal by your bed. If your mind is racing with worries or to-do lists, write them down. This simple act can help clear your mind and make it easier to relax.

Remember to be gentle with yourself. Rest may not come easily, but each moment of peace is a gift. Trust that God is watching over you, even in the darkest hours of the night.

Prayer

Lord, I struggle with restless nights and the anxiety that keeps me from sleeping. Please grant me Your peace and help me to rest in Your safety. Calm my mind and body, and fill my heart with Your serene presence. Amen.

Reflection

- What calming bedtime routines can you establish to help you find rest?

- How can you incorporate prayer and scripture into your night to seek God's peace?

_____

_____

_____

_____

_____

_____

FINANCIAL STRAIN

"And my God will meet all your needs according to the riches of his glory in Christ Jesus."

— PHILIPPIANS 4:19

One of the unexpected challenges of my cancer journey was the financial strain. The cost of treatments, medications, and missed work days added up quickly. It felt overwhelming, and I often worried about how I would manage it all.

During this time, Philippians 4:19 became a source of comfort and hope. The promise that God would meet all my needs according to His riches reminded me that I was not alone in this struggle. He knew my situation intimately and was fully capable of providing for me.

I began to see God's provision in ways I hadn't expected. Friends and family stepped in with financial support, sometimes surprising me with their generosity. I also discovered various resources and organizations specifically designed to help cancer patients with their financial burdens. Each gesture of support was a clear sign of God's care and provision.

Through prayer, I laid my financial worries before God, asking for His help and guidance. This act of surrender brought a sense of peace, allowing me to focus more on my healing journey. I learned that trusting in God's provision meant believing that He was already at work, even when I couldn't see the full picture.

This experience taught me that God's provision often comes through the kindness of others and the opportunities He places before us. By trusting Him with my financial concerns, I found that I could navigate this difficult path with greater confidence and less anxiety.

Prayer

Dear God, the financial strain of my journey feels overwhelming. Please provide for my needs and give me wisdom in managing my finances. Help me to trust in Your provision and to see the ways You are caring for me through others. Thank You for Your faithfulness and for meeting all my needs. Amen.

Reflection

- How has God provided for your needs in unexpected ways?

- What steps can you take to trust God more fully with your financial worries?

- *What do I want to remember about God's provision and care during moments of financial struggle?*

_____

_____

_____

MORE THAN A PATIENT

"For we are God's handiwork, created in Christ Jesus to do good works, which God prepared in advance for us to do."

— EPHESIANS 2:10

During your cancer journey, it can be easy to feel like your identity is consumed by your illness. Doctor's appointments, treatments, and rest dominate your schedule, and it can feel like there's little room for anything else. But remember, you are so much more than a patient.

You are God's handiwork, created with a unique purpose and equipped with gifts and talents that are not defined by your diagnosis. Take time to reconnect with the parts of yourself that bring joy and fulfillment. Whether it's a hobby you love, spending time with family, or volunteering in small ways, these activities can remind you of your greater purpose.

Consider how you can incorporate small acts of service into your routine. Maybe it's writing encouraging notes to others going through treatment, sharing your story to inspire hope, or finding creative ways to use your talents even in a limited capacity. These actions can help you feel connected to your purpose and remind you that you have so much to offer.

Balancing your roles means acknowledging the importance of your health while also embracing the other aspects of who you are. Trust that God has prepared good works for you to do, even in this season. Lean into His guidance and find ways to live out your purpose beyond your illness.

Prayer

Lord, help me to see myself as more than a patient. Remind me of the unique purpose You have for my life and the gifts You have given me. Show me how to balance my health needs with the other roles I cherish. Thank You for creating me with a purpose and for the good works You have prepared for me to do. Amen.

Reflection

• What activities or hobbies bring you joy and help you feel connected to your purpose?

• How can you incorporate small acts of service or creativity into your routine to remind yourself that you are more than a patient?

_____

_____

_____

_____

DATE

S   M   T   W   T   F   S

Facing Challenges Head-On

TRY SOMETHING NEW

Wear something that makes you feel good about yourself, like a favorite accessory or a new outfit.

What did you wear? How did it change your mood?

What I wore:

_____
_____

How I felt:

_____
_____
_____

LISTEN TO UPLIFTING MUSIC

Find a song or piece of music that lifts your spirits and listen to it. Let the music inspire you and bring a positive energy to your day.

What song did you choose? How did it affect your mood?

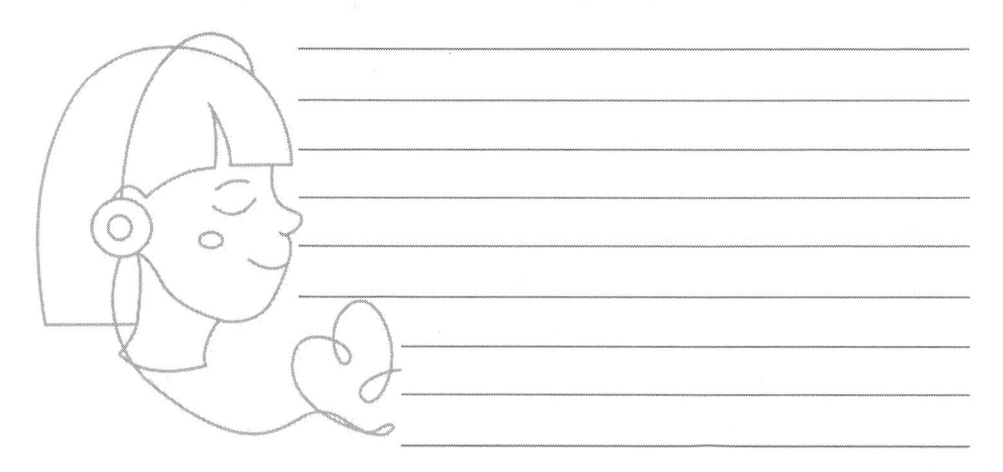

_____
_____
_____
_____
_____
_____
_____

AFFIRMATION BOARD

Write down a positive affirmation, such as "I am strong" or "I am loved," below. Look at it whenever you need encouragement.

How do you feel after?

You are beautiful and loved by God. Embrace your journey with confidence.

LIGHT THE PATH FOR ANOTHER WOMAN ON HER CANCER JOURNEY

"Carry each other's burdens, and in this way, you will fulfill the law of Christ."

— GALATIANS 6:2

Walking through the journey of cancer can be a challenging and lonely experience, but finding comfort and hope through this devotional can make a big difference. We hope these pages have been a source of strength, peace, and encouragement for you. Now, we have a special request.

Would you help someone you've never met, even if you never got credit for it?

Who is this person you ask? They are like you, or perhaps like you were at the beginning of this journey—seeking comfort, understanding, and hope during a difficult time.

Our mission is to provide spiritual and emotional support to every woman facing cancer. The only way for us to reach more women is by sharing the word, and your voice is powerful.

This is where you come in. Most people judge a book by its cover (and its reviews). So here's our ask on behalf of a struggling woman you've never met:

Please help that woman by leaving this book a review.

Your review costs no money and takes less than 60 seconds, but it could change another woman's life. Your review could help...

...one more woman find comfort during long, sleepless nights.
...one more reader feel understood and less alone in her journey.
...one more soul find peace and courage in the face of uncertainty.
...one more person discover the strength and support she needs.
...one more journey toward healing and hope.

To make this small but meaningful difference, all you have to do is **scan the QR code below:**

[Insert QR code]

[https://www.amazon.com/review/review-your-purchases/?asin=BOOKASIN]

Thank you from the bottom of our hearts.

Your biggest fan,

Biblical Teachings

Enduring the Journey

HALFWAY THERE

"Being confident of this, that he who began a good work in you will carry it on to completion until the day of Christ Jesus."

— PHILIPPIANS 1:6

When I reached the halfway point of my treatment, I felt a mix of relief and anxiety. There were days I wasn't sure I would make it this far. The journey had been long and difficult, filled with moments of doubt and pain. Yet, here I was, halfway through, and that was worth celebrating.

Reflecting on Philippians 1:6 brought me immense comfort. God, who began this journey with me, would carry it on to completion. He wasn't going to leave me halfway; He was committed to seeing me through.

To celebrate this milestone, I decided to do something special. I treated myself to a small gift, a reminder of my strength and perseverance. I also took time to thank those who had supported me—my family, friends, and medical team. Their encouragement and love had been a source of strength.

I realized that celebrating the halfway mark wasn't just about looking back; it was also about looking forward with hope. There was still a road ahead, but knowing that God was with me every step of the way gave me the courage to keep going.

If you're halfway through your treatment or any significant journey, take a moment to celebrate your progress. Thank God for His faithfulness and hold on to the promise that He will see you through to the end.

Prayer

Heavenly Father, thank You for being with me every step of this journey. As I reach this halfway point, I celebrate the progress made and the strength You have given me. Continue to carry me through to completion, and help me to trust in Your faithfulness. Amen.

Reflection

- How can you celebrate the progress you've made in your journey so far?

- What promises of God can you hold onto as you continue forward?

_____

_____

_____

_____

_____

TRUSTING THE PROCESS

"For I know the plans I have for you," declares the Lord, "plans to prosper you and not to harm you, plans to give you hope and a future."

— JEREMIAH 29:11

As you navigate through your treatment, it's natural to feel overwhelmed and uncertain. The side effects, the waiting, and the fear of the unknown can weigh heavily on your heart. But Jeremiah 29:11 reminds you that God has a plan for your life, a plan to give you hope and a future.

Trusting the process means believing that each step, no matter how difficult, is part of God's greater plan for your healing and restoration. It's about surrendering your fears and doubts to Him and trusting that He is in control.

When anxiety creeps in, find solace in the promise of Jeremiah 29:11. God knows the plans He has for you, and they are plans for your good. Even when the journey feels endless, trust that He is working everything together for your benefit.

Instead of focusing on the entire journey ahead, break it down into manageable parts. Start your day with a prayer or a moment of reflection, asking God for strength and guidance. Create small, achievable goals for the day, whether it's a walk outside, reading a chapter of a book, or calling a friend. Celebrate these small victories, as they are steps forward in your journey.

Seek out activities that bring you joy and peace. This might be listening to music, engaging in a hobby, or spending quiet time in nature. These moments can help ground you and remind you of the beauty and goodness still present in your life.

Trusting the process doesn't mean the journey will be easy, but it does mean you can have peace knowing that God is with you, guiding you towards a hopeful future.

Prayer

Lord, help me to trust the process and to believe in Your plan for my life. When I feel overwhelmed, remind me of Your promise to give me hope and a future. Strengthen my faith and help me to lean on You every step of the way. Amen.

Reflection

- How can you find ways to embrace the process of your journey?
- What steps can you take to trust God more fully with your future?

_____

_____

_____

BRIANNA'S STORY - DEALING WITH SETBACKS

"Consider it pure joy, my brothers and sisters, whenever you face trials of many kinds, because you know that the testing of your faith produces perseverance."

— JAMES 1:2-3

When Brianna received the news that her cancer had returned, it felt like a punch to the gut. She had been through so much already and was starting to feel hopeful about the future. This setback was a heavy blow, and she struggled to find the strength to face it.

Her friend Clara, who had experienced multiple recurrences, visited her one afternoon. *"I know how hard this is, Brianna," Clara said, taking her hand. "Each setback felt like the end for me too. But looking back, I see how it strengthened my faith and resilience. It's not easy, but God is with you, even in this."*

Encouraged by Clara's words, Brianna turned to James 1:2-3. The verse encouraged her to consider her trials as opportunities for growth. It was difficult to see the joy in such a painful situation, but she clung to the promise that her perseverance would be strengthened through this testing.

Brianna decided to take it one day at a time. She focused on the small victories and leaned heavily on prayer. She allowed herself to grieve but also looked for ways to find joy amidst the pain. Slowly, she began to see her setback not as a defeat, but as another step in her journey of faith.

Through her perseverance, Brianna discovered a deeper strength within herself and a closer relationship with God. Her story is a testament to the power of faith and the resilience that grows from trusting God through every trial.

Prayer

Dear God, setbacks are hard to face, and I struggle to find joy in these moments. Please give me the strength to persevere and to trust that You are with me in every trial. Help me to see these challenges as opportunities for growth and to lean on You for comfort and guidance. Amen.

Reflection

- How can you find ways to see setbacks as opportunities for growth?
- How can focusing on past victories help you face current challenges with renewed strength?

_____

_____

_____

_____

FINDING ENERGY TO KEEP GOING

"But those who hope in the Lord will renew their strength. They will soar on wings like eagles; they will run and not grow weary, they will walk and not be faint."

— ISAIAH 40:31

The fatigue hit me like a freight train. Some days, just getting out of bed felt like climbing a mountain. The treatments were taking a toll on my body and spirit, and I often wondered how I would find the energy to keep going. It was during one of these particularly tough days that I stumbled upon Isaiah 40:31.

The promise that those who hope in the Lord will renew their strength became my lifeline. I realized that my energy didn't have to come from my own reserves, which were often depleted. Instead, I could draw strength from God, who is limitless.

I began to start each day with a prayer, asking God to renew my strength. This simple act of surrender helped shift my focus from my limitations to His boundless power. On days when I felt particularly drained, I made a conscious effort to listen to my body and give myself grace. Rest was no longer a sign of weakness but a necessary part of my healing.

Finding energy also meant discovering small moments of joy and hope. I started to keep a journal of these moments—like the warmth of the sun on my face, the sound of birds singing outside my window, or the comfort of a loved one's embrace. One day, a friend brought me a small bouquet of flowers. The vibrant colors and delicate fragrance brought a smile to my face and a lift to my spirit. It was in these tiny, seemingly insignificant moments that I found the motivation to keep going.

One evening, I sat quietly in my room, the soft glow of a candle flickering nearby. I opened my Bible and read Isaiah 40:31 again, letting the words wash over me. I could almost feel the weight lifting from my shoulders as I placed my trust in God's promise.

If you're struggling to find the energy to keep going, remember that you don't have to do it alone. Place your hope in the Lord, and let Him renew your strength each day. Embrace the small moments of joy and let them be reminders of God's unwavering presence in your life.

Prayer

Heavenly Father, I feel so drained and weary. Please renew my strength and help me to find energy in You. Guide me to rest when I need it and to draw joy from the small moments in life. Thank You for being my source of strength and hope. Amen.

Reflection

- How can you draw strength from God when you feel exhausted?

- What small moments of joy can you find to renew your energy?

- *What do I want to remember about my own resilience and ability to find strength, even in difficult times?*

HOPE ON HARD DAYS

"May the God of hope fill you with all joy and peace as you trust in him, so that you may overflow with hope by the power of the Holy Spirit."

— ROMANS 15:13

There are days when everything feels like an uphill battle. The treatment side effects, the endless appointments, and the emotional toll can make it hard to see any light at the end of the tunnel. But even on the hardest days, hope is not out of reach.

Romans 15:13 reminds you that God is the source of all hope. He wants to fill you with joy and peace, even in the midst of your struggles. Trusting in Him allows the power of the Holy Spirit to work within you, overflowing your heart with hope.

On those tough days, take a moment to pause and breathe. Turn your worries and fears over to God in prayer. Ask Him to fill you with His hope and peace. It might help to keep a gratitude journal, where you write down even the smallest things you are thankful for. This practice can shift your focus from what's going wrong to the blessings that still surround you.

Connect with others who uplift you. Sometimes, a simple conversation with a friend or family member can remind you that you are not alone. Their encouragement and support can be a beacon of hope on the darkest days.

Remember, it's okay to have hard days. But even in those moments, God's hope is available to you. Trust in Him, and let His joy and peace overflow in your heart.

Prayer

Lord, on my hardest days, fill me with Your hope and peace. Help me to trust in You and to see the blessings around me. Let Your Holy Spirit overflow in my heart, giving me the strength and encouragement I need. Amen.

Reflection

- How can you seek God's hope and peace on your hardest days?
- What memories or positive experiences can you reflect on to uplift your spirits?

ALLOWING YOURSELF TO BE HUMAN

"For we do not have a high priest who is unable to empathize with our weaknesses, but we have one who has been tempted in every way, just as we are—yet he did not sin."

— HEBREWS 4:15

As you journey through treatment, it's important to remember that it's okay to be human. There will be days when you feel strong and days when you feel utterly defeated. Jesus understands your weaknesses and empathizes with your struggles.

Hebrews 4:15 reminds us that Jesus experienced human emotions and temptations. He understands what it means to feel pain, fear, and sorrow. Knowing this can bring great comfort because it means that you don't have to hide your feelings from Him. You can bring your raw, honest emotions to Jesus, and He will understand.

Give yourself permission to feel. It's okay to cry, to feel frustrated, or to simply have a bad day. Acknowledge your emotions and bring them to God in prayer. Allow His empathy and love to comfort you.

Remember that being human also means recognizing your limits. You don't have to be strong all the time. Lean on your support network, ask for help when you need it, and take time to rest.

Allowing yourself to be human is not a sign of weakness; it's a testament to your resilience and faith. Embrace your humanity, knowing that Jesus walks with you through every high and low.

Prayer

Dear Jesus, thank You for understanding my weaknesses and for walking with me through every struggle. Help me to be honest about my feelings and to bring them to You. Give me the strength to embrace my humanity and to find comfort in Your empathy and love. Amen.

Reflection

- How can you be more honest about your emotions with yourself and with God?

- How can acknowledging your own limitations lead to personal growth and healing?

_____

_____

_____

_____

_____

_____

DIVINE STRENGTH

"The Lord is my strength and my song; he has given me victory."

— EXODUS 15:2

When the weight of my treatment journey feels too heavy to bear, I find myself turning to Exodus 15:2. This verse has become a source of incredible strength and encouragement for me. It reminds me that I am not alone in this battle; I have divine strength to rely on.

There have been days when I felt like I couldn't take another step. The physical pain, the emotional exhaustion, and the constant challenges seemed insurmountable. In those moments, I would close my eyes and repeat, *"The Lord is my strength and my song; he has given me victory."* This simple act of faith would renew my spirit and give me the courage to keep going.

Relying on divine strength means acknowledging that I don't have to do it all on my own. God's power is made perfect in my weakness. When I feel like giving up, I turn to Him in prayer, asking for the strength to face each new day. He has never failed to provide me with the resilience and determination I need.

I also find strength in sharing my journey with others. Talking about my struggles and victories with friends, family, or support groups helps me feel connected and less isolated. Their prayers and encouragement are a reminder of God's love and support.

If you're feeling overwhelmed, remember that you don't have to carry this burden alone. Rely on the divine strength that God offers, and trust that He will give you the power to overcome any obstacle.

Prayer

Lord, thank You for the strength You provide. Help me to rely on Your power and not my own. When I feel weak, remind me that You are my strength and my song, and You have given me victory. Give me the courage to face each day with faith and resilience. Amen.

Reflection

- How can you rely more on God's strength in your daily challenges?
- What past experiences can you reflect on to see how God has provided for you?

_____

_____

_____

_____

_____

WORDS TO LIFT YOUR SPIRIT

"The Lord is near to the brokenhearted and saves the crushed in spirit."

— PSALM 34:18

Some days, the weight of the world feels unbearable, and it's easy to feel crushed in spirit. During these times, the right words can lift you up and bring a sense of peace. Psalm 34:18 reminds you that the Lord is near to the brokenhearted and saves those who are crushed in spirit.

When you feel overwhelmed, surround yourself with words of encouragement. Start by writing down your favorite Bible verses and placing them where you can see them throughout the day—on your bathroom mirror, your refrigerator, or even your phone's lock screen. These reminders of God's love and presence can lift your spirit when you need it most.

Consider keeping a journal where you write down positive affirmations and prayers. Each morning, take a few moments to read these words and meditate on their meaning. Speak them aloud, letting the truth of God's promises sink deep into your heart.

Reach out to friends and family members who can offer words of encouragement and prayer. Sometimes, hearing a comforting voice or receiving a heartfelt message can make a significant difference. Let their support and love remind you that you are not alone in this journey.

Finally, listen to uplifting music or podcasts that speak to your soul. Let the melodies and words wash over you, bringing a sense of calm and hope.

Remember, the Lord is always near, ready to lift your spirit and save you in times of need. Embrace His presence and let His words fill you with peace and strength.

Prayer

Lord, I often feel overwhelmed and crushed in spirit. Please lift me up with Your words of comfort and love. Surround me with encouraging voices and reminders of Your presence. Help me to find peace and strength in Your promises. Amen.

Reflection

- How can you incorporate encouraging words and affirmations into your daily routine?

- Who in your life can you reach out to for support and uplifting conversation?

- *What do I want to remember about how words of encouragement have helped me through tough moments?*

OLIVIA'S STORY - STRENGTH IN NUMBERS

"For where two or three gather in my name, there am I with them."

— MATTHEW 18:20

When Olivia was first diagnosed with cancer, she felt an overwhelming sense of isolation. The journey ahead seemed lonely and daunting. One day, her oncologist suggested she join a support group for women undergoing similar treatments. Skeptical but desperate for connection, Olivia decided to attend.

During her first meeting, she met Sadie, who had been battling cancer for several years. Sadie shared her experience with a warm smile, *"I thought I had to be strong on my own, but I learned that true strength comes from leaning on others. We are stronger together."*

Olivia was moved by Sadie's words. As the group continued to meet, she found herself opening up about her fears and struggles. The women in the group shared their stories, offered advice, and most importantly, prayed together. Olivia felt a profound sense of God's presence in those gatherings, a tangible reminder of Matthew 18:20: *"For where two or three gather in my name, there am I with them."*

One day, Olivia shared a particularly difficult experience she had during treatment. The group responded with overwhelming support and love. Sadie hugged her and said, *"We're here for you, Olivia. You don't have to go through this alone."*

Through these meetings, Olivia discovered the power of community. The shared prayers, encouragement, and understanding turned her isolation into a shared journey of faith and resilience. The strength she found in numbers not only helped her endure her treatment but also deepened her trust in God's provision through others.

Olivia's story is a testament to the strength found in community. When we gather with others in faith, we experience God's presence in profound ways. Together, we can endure, thrive, and support one another through even the toughest challenges.

Prayer

Dear God, thank You for the strength that comes from community. Help me to seek out and lean on others who understand my journey. May we find comfort and resilience in Your presence as we gather together. Amen.

Reflection

- How can you connect with others who share similar experiences to find strength and support?

- What role does community play in your journey of faith and healing?

WALKING BY FAITH

"For we walk by faith, not by sight."

— 2 CORINTHIANS 5:7

The path of cancer treatment is often filled with uncertainties. The future may seem unclear, and the journey can be daunting. Yet, in 2 Corinthians 5:7, we are reminded to walk by faith, not by sight. This verse encourages you to trust in God's guidance, even when you cannot see the way forward.

Walking by faith means relying on God's promises rather than your circumstances. It's about believing that He is leading you, even through the darkest valleys. Each step you take is a testament to your trust in His plan and His love for you.

When doubt and fear creep in, turn to prayer. Ask God to strengthen your faith and to help you see beyond your current situation. Spend time in His Word, drawing comfort from the stories of those who have walked by faith before you. Let their journeys inspire you to keep moving forward, even when the path is unclear.

Surround yourself with a community of believers who can support and encourage you. Their faith and prayers can bolster your own, reminding you that you are not walking this journey alone. Together, you can find the strength to trust in God's promises and to keep moving forward in faith.

Remember, walking by faith doesn't mean you will never feel fear or doubt. It means choosing to trust God in spite of those feelings, knowing that He is with you every step of the way.

Prayer

Lord, help me to walk by faith and not by sight. Strengthen my trust in Your promises, and guide me through the uncertainties of this journey. Surround me with a community that supports and encourages my faith. Thank You for leading me, even when I cannot see the way forward. Amen.

Reflection

- How can you practice walking by faith in your daily life?
- What are some examples of times when walking by faith has positively impacted your life?

_____

_____

_____

_____

_____

DATE

S M T W T F S

Enduring the Journey

CELEBRATE SMALL WINS

When you reach a milestone, celebrate it with a small treat or activity you enjoy. What did you celebrate? How did you celebrate it?

What I celebrated:

_____
_____

How I celebrated:

_____
_____
_____

REFLECT ON YOUR PROGRESS

Take a few moments to reflect on how far you've come since starting your journey. What achievements, big or small, are you proud of?

List at least three achievements:

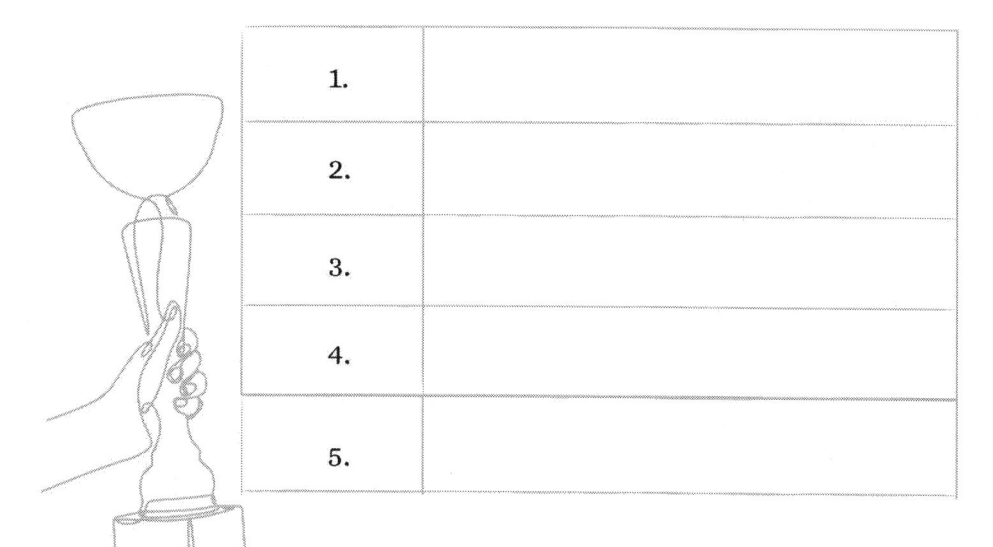

1.	
2.	
3.	
4.	
5.	

HOPEFUL COLLAGE

Cut out images and words from that represent hope and your future aspirations. Arrange them into a collage.

What does your collage represent?

_____
_____
_____
_____

Celebrate your progress, practice kindness, and keep hope alive as you continue your journey.

Nearing the Finish Line

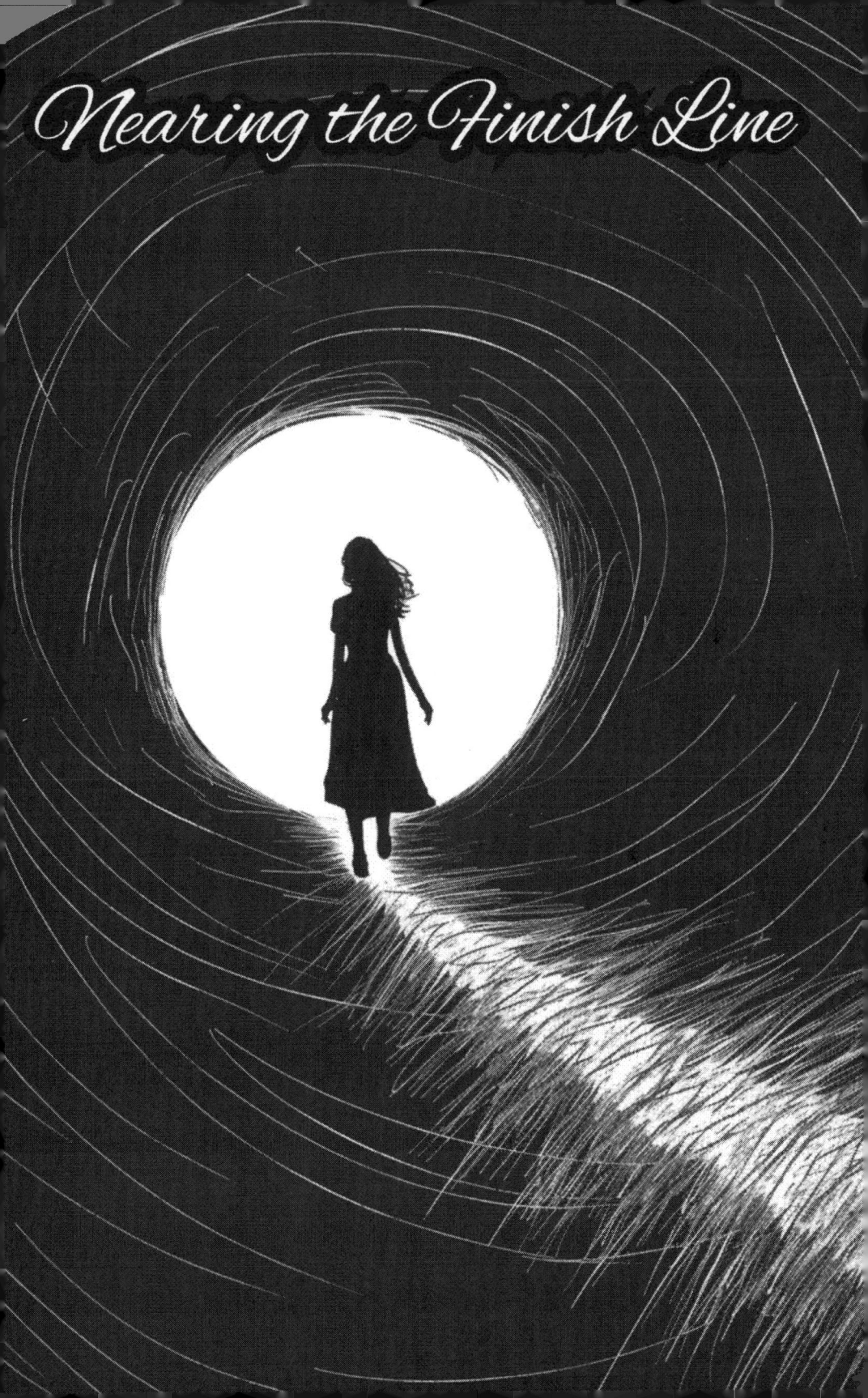

SEEING THE LIGHT

"The light shines in the darkness, and the darkness has not overcome it."

— JOHN 1:5

As I approached the end of my treatment, I felt a mixture of relief, excitement, and anxiety. The journey had been long and grueling, filled with moments of doubt and fear. But now, I could finally see the light at the end of the tunnel. The words of John 1:5 resonated deeply with me: *"The light shines in the darkness, and the darkness has not overcome it."*

I began to reflect on the past months. Each treatment session, each side effect, each sleepless night—they all seemed to blur together. But through it all, there was a constant presence of hope and light. God had been my beacon, guiding me through the darkest times.

One day, during a particularly challenging treatment, a nurse looked at me and said, *"You're almost there. Just a little more to go."* Her words were simple, but they sparked a renewed sense of determination in me. I realized that this journey, with all its hardships, was drawing to a close. I could feel the warmth of the light breaking through the darkness.

I started to focus on the small victories. Each day that brought me closer to the end of treatment was a day worth celebrating. I allowed myself to dream about the future, to envision a life beyond cancer. These thoughts filled me with hope and strength.

As I approached the final stages of my treatment, I held tightly to the promise that the light would overcome the darkness. God's presence had been my strength, and I knew He would continue to guide me as I neared the finish line.

Prayer

Heavenly Father, thank You for being my light in the darkness. As I approach the end of my treatment, fill me with hope and strength. Help me to see the light breaking through and to trust in Your continued guidance. Amen.

Reflection

- How has God's light guided you through your treatment journey?

- What small victories can you celebrate as you approach the end of your treatment?

_____

_____

_____

_____

PREPARING FOR THE NEXT STEPS

"For I know the plans I have for you," declares the Lord, "plans to prosper you and not to harm you, plans to give you hope and a future."

— JEREMIAH 29:11

As your treatment journey draws to a close, it's natural to feel a mixture of relief and uncertainty about the future. You've come so far, but what comes next? Jeremiah 29:11 offers a comforting reminder that God has a plan for your life—a plan to give you hope and a future.

You might have received plenty of advice, well-meaning but sometimes overwhelming. People often share their experiences, recommend miracle cures, or offer help in various ways. But as time goes on, these offers often fade, and you might feel like you're facing the future alone. If you're feeling deserted, know that God is always with you. He has a plan for you, a plan to give you hope and a future.

Preparing for the next steps involves both practical and emotional readiness. Take time to meet with your medical team to discuss follow-up care and any ongoing treatments or check-ups. Understanding what to expect can help ease some of the anxiety about the unknown.

Emotionally, it's important to acknowledge the journey you've been on. Give yourself permission to feel whatever comes up—whether it's relief, joy, fear, or a mixture of emotions. Each feeling is valid and part of your healing process.

Consider creating a new routine that incorporates both rest and activities that bring you joy. Now is the time to rediscover hobbies and interests that may have been put on hold. Spend time in prayer and reflection, asking God to guide you as you step into this new phase of life.

Surround yourself with a supportive community. Friends, family, and support groups can provide encouragement and understanding as you transition from treatment to recovery. Lean on them and share your hopes and fears.

Remember, God's plans for you are good. Trust in His guidance as you prepare for the next steps, knowing that He is with you every step of the way.

Prayer

Lord, thank You for bringing me through this treatment journey. As I prepare for the next steps, guide me with Your wisdom and peace. Help me to trust in Your plans for my future and to find joy and hope in this new phase of life. Amen.

Reflection

- How can you prepare both practically and emotionally for the next steps after treatment?

- What activities and routines can you incorporate to help you transition into recovery?

- *What do I want to remember about the strength and growth I've gained as I move into the next chapter of recovery?*

AMELIA'S STORY - PUSHING THROUGH THE LAST STAGES

"I have fought the good fight, I have finished the race, I have kept the faith."

— 2 TIMOTHY 4:7

Cancer has a way of making time feel like it's stretching on endlessly, especially as you near the end of treatment. The final stages can test your endurance and spirit in ways you never anticipated. Each day feels like an uphill battle, but every step forward is a testament to your strength and faith.

I've always believed in being prepared for life's challenges—whether it was carrying an umbrella when it looked like rain or keeping extra gifts ready for unexpected occasions. But nothing could have prepared me for the exhaustion and emotional toll of cancer treatment. The last few treatments seemed to stretch on forever, testing my endurance and spirit.

Amelia had reached the final stages of her treatment, but the journey had been anything but easy. The last few treatments seemed to stretch on forever, testing her endurance and spirit. There were days when she felt like giving up, but she held onto the words of 2 Timothy 4:7: *"I have fought the good fight, I have finished the race, I have kept the faith."*

During a particularly tough week, Amelia attended her support group. *"I'm so close to the end, but I feel like I have nothing left to give,"* she confessed to the group. Her friends, who had become like family, offered her encouragement and love.

"I remember feeling the same way," said Josephine, a survivor who had completed her treatment the previous year. *"But just when I thought I couldn't take another step, I found strength in my faith and in the support of those around me. You've come this far, Amelia. Keep pushing through."*

Amelia took these words to heart. She leaned on her faith, praying for the strength to endure the final treatments. She also allowed herself to lean on her support system, accepting help and encouragement from her friends and family.

As the days passed, Amelia began to see the light at the end of the tunnel. She marked each completed treatment with a small celebration, acknowledging her perseverance and the progress she had made. The words of 2 Timothy 4:7 became a mantra, reminding her that she was fighting the good fight and keeping the faith.

Finally, the day came when Amelia finished her last treatment. Tears of joy and relief filled her eyes as she realized she had made it through. The journey had been long and hard, but she had finished the race with faith and strength.

Amelia's story is a powerful reminder that even in the hardest stages, God provides the strength to endure. With faith and the support of others, you can push through and finish your race.

Prayer

Dear God, as I push through the last stages of my treatment, give me the strength and endurance I need. Help me to lean on my faith and the support of those around me. Thank You for guiding me through this journey and helping me to finish the race. Amen.

Reflection

- What scripture verses provide you with hope and motivation during this time?

- What positive affirmations can you repeat to yourself to maintain a hopeful outlook?

_____

_____

_____

_____

_____

_____

_____

_____

_____

_____

_____

_____

_____

_____

FAITH IN THE FINISH LINE

"Being confident of this, that he who began a good work in you will carry it on to completion until the day of Christ Jesus."

— PHILIPPIANS 1:6

As I neared the end of my treatment, the finish line finally came into view. The journey had been long, filled with moments of doubt and despair, but also with glimmers of hope and faith. Philippians 1:6 became my anchor: *"Being confident of this, that he who began a good work in you will carry it on to completion until the day of Christ Jesus."*

Every step of the way, I felt God's presence guiding me, giving me the strength to keep going. There were days when I questioned if I could make it to the end, but each time, God reminded me that He had begun this good work in me and would see it through.

I remember sitting in the waiting room on my last day of treatment, feeling a rush of emotions. Relief, gratitude, and a sense of accomplishment washed over me. I reflected on the countless prayers, the support from loved ones, and the small victories that had carried me through. It was my faith that sustained me, reminding me that God's promises are true and that He would carry me to completion.

Reaching the finish line doesn't mean the journey is over; it's a new beginning. My faith in God's promises and His continuous work in my life has given me the courage to face each new day with hope and strength. Trusting in His plan, I move forward, confident that He will continue to guide me.

Prayer

Heavenly Father, thank You for carrying me through this journey and for being my constant source of strength. As I reach the finish line, help me to trust in Your continued work in my life. Fill me with hope and courage as I step into this new chapter. Amen.

Reflection

- How has your faith sustained you throughout your treatment?
- What does reaching the finish line mean to you, and how can you trust in God's continued guidance?

GOD'S PROMISES

"But I will restore you to health and heal your wounds,' declares the Lord."

— JEREMIAH 30:17

As you near the end of your treatment, it's important to hold on to the promises of God's healing. Jeremiah 30:17 offers a powerful reminder: *"But I will restore you to health and heal your wounds,' declares the Lord."*

God's promises are not just about physical healing but encompass emotional and spiritual restoration as well. Throughout your journey, you've faced numerous challenges, and each step has been a testament to your resilience and faith.

Reflect on the ways God has already begun to heal you. Perhaps it's the support of friends and family, the small moments of joy amidst the struggle, or the inner strength you've discovered. These are all signs of God's healing hand at work in your life.

Take time to pray and meditate on His promises. Trust that He is with you, even when the path seems uncertain. His healing may come in different forms, and His timing may not always align with ours, but His promises are true and steadfast.

As you transition from treatment to recovery, lean into His word and let His promises of healing and restoration fill you with hope. Remember, you are not alone in this journey. God is with you, guiding and healing you every step of the way.

Prayer

Lord, thank You for Your promises of healing and restoration. Help me to trust in Your timing and to see the signs of Your healing in my life. Fill me with hope and peace as I continue this journey with You. Amen.

Reflection

- How have you experienced God's healing in your life so far?
- What promises of God can you hold on to as you transition to recovery?
- What do I want to remember about how God has kept His promises during my recovery?

_____

_____

_____

_____

_____

_____

CAROLINE'S STORY - REFLECTING ON THE JOURNEY

"The Lord has done great things for us, and we are filled with joy."

— PSALM 126:3

Caroline sat quietly in her favorite chair, a warm cup of tea in her hands. The final treatment was behind her, and she felt a mix of relief and uncertainty about what lay ahead. As she reflected on the journey, she couldn't help but feel a deep sense of gratitude for all the ways God had carried her through.

Caroline's journey had been filled with challenges, but it had also been marked by moments of profound grace and love. She recalled the nights she spent in prayer, the encouragement from friends and family, and the small victories that kept her going. Through it all, she felt God's presence, guiding her and giving her strength.

One evening, during a support group meeting, she shared her reflections with the group. *"Looking back, I see how far I've come and how much I've grown,"* she said. *"There were times I wanted to give up, but

God's love and the support of all of you kept me going. The Lord has done great things for us, and we are filled with joy."

Paula, a fellow survivor, nodded in agreement. *"It's incredible to see the transformation in each of us. God's faithfulness is evident in our stories, and we can move forward with hope and joy."*

Reflecting on the journey allowed Caroline to see the bigger picture. It wasn't just about the struggle; it was about the growth, the resilience, and the faith that had blossomed through adversity. The words of Psalm 126:3 echoed in her heart: *"The Lord has done great things for us, and we are filled with joy."*

Caroline's story is a powerful reminder to take time to reflect on your own journey. Acknowledge the hardships, but also celebrate the victories and the growth. God has been with you every step of the way, and His great works fill us with joy.

Prayer

Dear God, as I reflect on my journey, I am filled with gratitude for Your presence and guidance. Thank You for the strength and growth You have given me. Help me to see the great things You have done in my life and to move forward with joy and hope. Amen.

Reflection

- How has reflecting on your journey helped you see God's work in your life?
- What moments of grace and growth can you celebrate as you move forward?

JOY IN SMALL MOMENTS

"This is the day that the Lord has made; let us rejoice and be glad in it."

— PSALM 118:24

The journey through cancer treatment taught me to find joy in the small moments. There were days when the big picture felt overwhelming, but the small blessings carried me through. Psalm 118:24 became a daily reminder to rejoice in each day, no matter how challenging it might be: *"This is the day that the Lord has made; let us rejoice and be glad in it."*

I remember one morning, early in my treatment, when I woke up feeling particularly low. The side effects were hitting hard, and I struggled to find a reason to get out of bed. Then, I heard the birds singing outside my window. Their cheerful melodies reminded me of the beauty and simplicity of life. That small moment brought a smile to my face and lifted my spirits.

Throughout my journey, I learned to cherish these small moments. A kind word from a nurse, a delicious meal shared with a friend, or a quiet evening spent with a good book—each of these moments became a source of joy and strength.

Celebrating the small victories also became important. Completing a treatment session, enjoying a day without nausea, or simply feeling a bit more energetic were all reasons to be grateful. These moments of joy helped me stay focused on the positive and reminded me that, even in the midst of struggle, there is always something to be thankful for.

As I move forward, I continue to seek out and celebrate these small moments of joy. They remind me of God's presence in my life and the countless blessings He provides each day.

Prayer

Dear Lord, thank You for the small moments of joy that brighten my days. Help me to see and celebrate these blessings, even in the midst of challenges. Fill my heart with gratitude and remind me of Your constant presence. Amen.

Reflection

- What small moments of joy can you celebrate today?
- How can focusing on these moments help you stay positive and grateful?

_____

_____

_____

_____

BUILDING NEW DREAMS

"Therefore, if anyone is in Christ, the new creation has come: The old has gone, the new is here!"

— 2 CORINTHIANS 5:17

As you transition into life beyond cancer, it's time to start building new dreams. The journey you've been on has changed you in profound ways, and now you have the opportunity to create a future that reflects your new perspective. 2 Corinthians 5:17 reminds you of this transformation: *"Therefore, if anyone is in Christ, the new creation has come: The old has gone, the new is here!"*

Building new dreams begins with reflecting on what truly matters to you. The experience of cancer may have shifted your priorities, highlighting what is most important in your life. Take time to consider your passions, values, and aspirations. What excites you? What gives you a sense of purpose?

Start by setting small, achievable goals. These can be steps towards larger dreams, helping you build momentum and confidence. Perhaps it's learning a new skill, rekindling a hobby, or volunteering for a cause close to your heart. Each small step is a building block towards your new future.

It's also essential to lean on your faith during this time. Pray for guidance and clarity as you envision your new dreams. Trust that God is leading you and that His plans for you are filled with hope and promise.

Remember, it's okay to dream big. Your journey has shown you that you are capable of overcoming great challenges, and now you can channel that strength into creating a vibrant, fulfilling future. Embrace this new chapter with an open heart and a spirit of adventure.

Prayer

Lord, thank You for the new creation You have made me. As I build new dreams, guide my steps and fill me with hope and courage. Help me to trust in Your plans and to embrace this new chapter with joy. Amen.

Reflection

- What new dreams and goals are you excited to pursue?

- How can your faith guide you as you build this new chapter of your life?

- What do I want to remember about this moment as I move forward in building new dreams?

_____

_____

_____

SEEKING GUIDANCE FOR THE NEXT PHASE

"Your word is a lamp for my feet, a light on my path."

— PSALM 119:105

The end of cancer treatment marks the beginning of a new phase, filled with its own set of challenges and opportunities. As I stepped into this new chapter, I found myself seeking guidance more than ever. Psalm 119:105 became a cornerstone for me: *"Your word is a lamp for my feet, a light on my path."*

Throughout my treatment, I had leaned heavily on prayer and scripture, finding comfort and direction in God's word. Now, as I looked towards the future, I continued to seek His guidance. I needed clarity on how to navigate this new terrain, how to rebuild my life, and how to maintain my health and well-being.

I spent more time in prayer, asking God to reveal His plans for me and to show me the next steps. I found solace in the stillness, listening for His voice and trusting that He would lead me. There were days of uncertainty, but I held onto the promise that God's word would illuminate my path.

I also sought counsel from trusted friends, family, and spiritual advisors. Their wisdom and support provided additional clarity and encouragement. They reminded me that it's okay to take things one step at a time and that God's guidance often comes through the people He places in our lives.

As I moved forward, I embraced the new phase with an open heart, ready to follow wherever God led me. I learned to trust in His timing and His plan, knowing that He had brought me this far and would continue to guide me.

Prayer

Heavenly Father, as I step into this new phase, I seek Your guidance and wisdom. Illuminate my path and show me the way forward. Help me to trust in Your word and to lean on the support of those around me. Thank You for being my constant guide and light. Amen.

Reflection

- How can you seek God's guidance in this new phase of your life?
- Who can you turn to for wisdom and support as you navigate this new chapter?

_____

_____

_____

_____

_____

DATE	
S M T W T F S	

Approaching the End of Treatment

REFLECT ON STRENGTH

Think about three times you showed strength during your journey.

Strength Moment 1	
Strength Moment 2	
Strength Moment 3	

WRITE A LETTER TO YOUR FUTURE SELF

Write a short letter to your future self, reflecting on what you've learned and what you hope to remember as you move forward.

Hi future self,

_____

_____

_____

_____

_____

_____

_____

_____

_____

PLAN A CELEBRATION

Plan a small celebration to mark the end of your treatment, whether it's a special meal, gathering with loved ones, or a quiet moment of reflection.

What will you do to celebrate?

_____
_____
_____
_____
_____

As you near the end of treatment, remember your strength and spread kindness. Look forward with hope.

Living Beyond Cancer

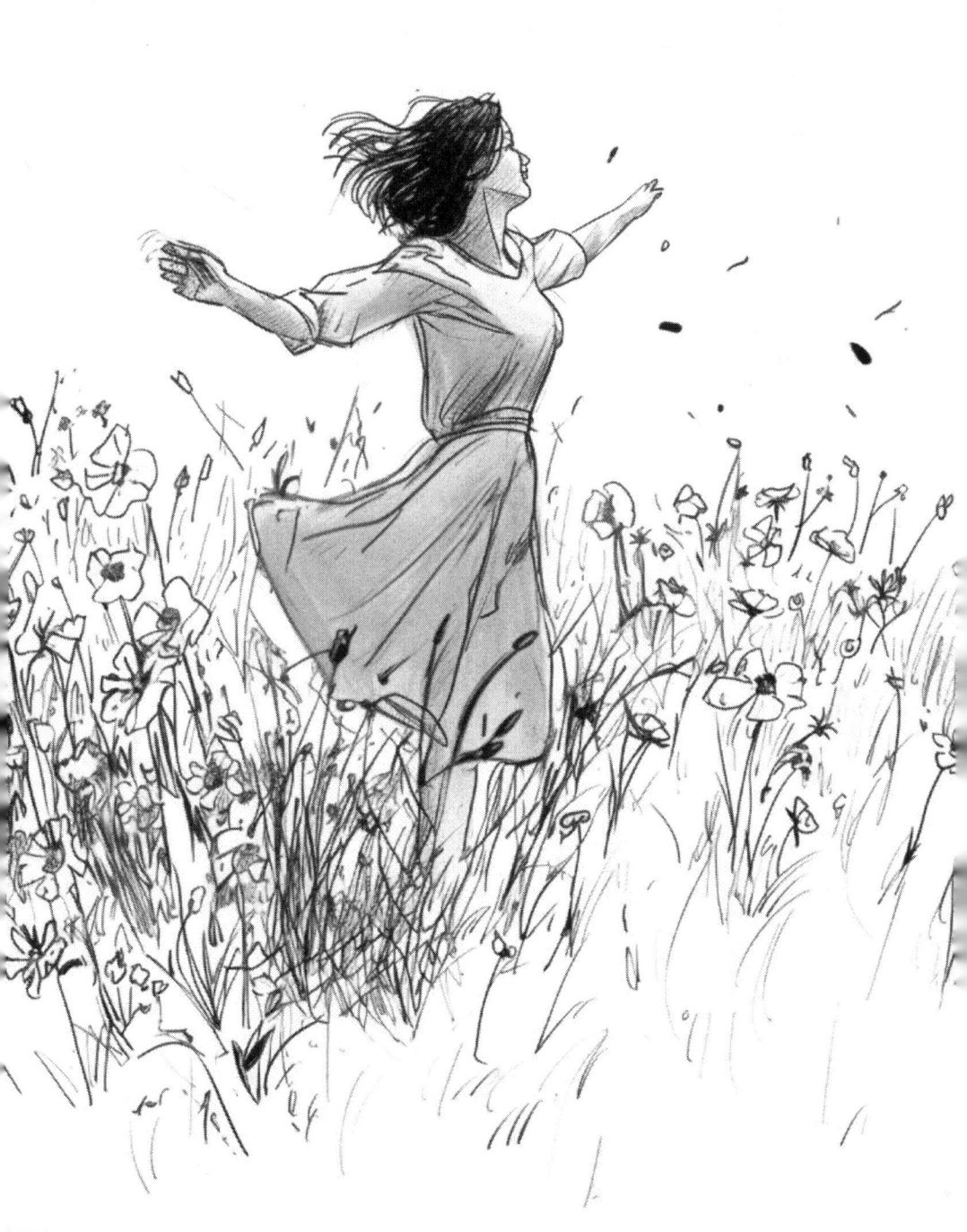

ADJUSTING TO LIFE AFTER TREATMENT

"For I am about to do something new. See, I have already begun! Do you not see it? I will make a pathway through the wilderness. I will create rivers in the dry wasteland."

— ISAIAH 43:19

The end of your cancer treatment marks the beginning of a new chapter in your life. This transition can be both exciting and overwhelming as you adjust to a life that is no longer dominated by treatments and hospital visits. Isaiah 43:19 reminds you that God is doing something new in your life, creating pathways through the wilderness and bringing rivers to the dry wasteland.

Adjusting to life after treatment means finding a new normal. It's okay to feel a mix of emotions—relief, joy, anxiety, and even sadness. Give yourself permission to experience these feelings and to take things one step at a time.

There may be days when you feel uncertain or lost, wondering how to move forward. Remember that it's natural to feel this way. You've been through a transformative journey, and it will take time to find your footing again. Embrace the process with patience and grace.

Prayer

Lord, as I adjust to life after treatment, help me to see the new things You are doing in my life. Guide me as I establish a routine that supports my well-being and helps me to embrace this new chapter. Thank You for being with me every step of the way. Amen.

Reflection

- What new routines and activities can you incorporate into your life after treatment?
- How can you continue to seek God's guidance and presence in this new chapter?

DEALING WITH FEAR OF RECURRENCE

"When I am afraid, I put my trust in you."

— PSALM 56:3

The end of treatment is a significant milestone, but it also brings a new set of challenges, including the fear of recurrence. This fear can be overwhelming, making it difficult to fully enjoy the newfound freedom and relief. Psalm 56:3 offers comfort in these moments: *"When I am afraid, I put my trust in you."*

As I finished my treatment, the fear of recurrence loomed large in my mind. Every ache and pain sparked anxiety, and I found myself constantly worrying about the future. It was during one of these anxious moments that I turned to Psalm 56:3. The simple act of putting my trust in God helped to calm my fears and bring a sense of peace.

Dealing with the fear of recurrence involves acknowledging your feelings and finding healthy ways to cope with them. Here are a few strategies that helped me:

1. **Stay Connected to Your Medical Team:** Regular check-ups and open communication with your healthcare providers can help alleviate some of your fears. They can provide reassurance and monitor your health closely.
2. **Lean on Your Support System:** Talk to friends, family, or support groups about your fears. Sharing your feelings can reduce the burden and help you feel understood and supported.
3. **Practice Mindfulness and Relaxation Techniques:** Techniques such as deep breathing, meditation, and yoga can help calm your mind and reduce anxiety.
4. **Focus on the Present:** Instead of worrying about what might happen, try to focus on the present moment. Enjoy the small joys of daily life and take things one day at a time.
5. **Trust in God's Plan:** Remind yourself of God's promises and His presence in your life. When fear arises, turn to Him in prayer, asking for peace and strength.

Remember, it's natural to feel afraid, but you don't have to face these fears alone. Put your trust in God, knowing that He is with you every step of the way, providing comfort and peace.

Prayer

Lord, when I am afraid, help me to put my trust in You. Calm my fears and fill me with Your peace. Guide me as I navigate this new phase of life and help me to trust in Your plan for my future. Amen.

Reflection

- How can you cope with the fear of recurrence in healthy ways?

BIBLICAL TEACHINGS

- What strategies can help you to focus on the present and trust in God's plan?

LAURA'S STORY - CONTINUING SELF-CARE

"Come to me, all you who are weary and burdened, and I will give you rest."

— MATTHEW 11:28

After finishing her cancer treatment, Laura found herself at a crossroads. The relentless pace of medical appointments and treatments had ceased, leaving a void she wasn't sure how to fill. It was then that she realized the importance of continuing self-care, not just for her body, but for her mind and spirit as well.

Laura remembered the words of Matthew 11:28: *"Come to me, all you who are weary and burdened, and I will give you rest."* She had felt weariness in every part of her being, and now she was learning to seek the rest and peace that only God could provide.

Laura started small. She began by setting aside a few minutes each day for prayer and meditation, allowing herself to connect with God and find solace in His presence. She also made time for activities that brought her joy, whether it was reading a good book, taking a walk in nature, or spending quality time with loved ones.

One day, Laura shared her journey with her support group. *"I've learned that self-care isn't just about the physical aspect,"* she said. *"It's about nurturing our entire being—body, mind, and spirit. And it's something we need to prioritize even after treatment ends."*

Her words resonated deeply with the group. They realized that self-care was a continuous journey, one that required intentionality and commitment. It was about finding balance, seeking rest in God's presence, and embracing activities that nourished their souls.

Laura's story reminds us that self-care is an ongoing process. It's about finding moments of rest and peace, and allowing ourselves to be replenished by God's love and grace. As you continue on your journey, remember to prioritize self-care in all its forms and to seek the rest that God so graciously offers.

Prayer

Dear God, thank You for the gift of rest and self-care. Help me to prioritize my well-being and to seek Your presence in moments of weariness. Guide me as I continue to nurture my body, mind, and spirit. Amen.

Reflection

- How can you incorporate self-care into your daily routine?
- What activities bring you joy and help you feel replenished?

_____

_____

_____

_____

RECOVERING MENTALLY AND SPIRITUALLY

"The Lord is close to the brokenhearted and saves those who are crushed in spirit."

— PSALM 34:18

As you transition to life beyond cancer, it's important to focus on recovering both mentally and spiritually. The journey you've been on has taken a toll not just on your body, but on your mind and spirit as well. Psalm 34:18 offers a comforting reminder: *"The Lord is close to the brokenhearted and saves those who are crushed in spirit."*

Recovering mentally means acknowledging the emotional impact of your experience. It's okay to feel a range of emotions, from relief and joy to anxiety and sadness. Allow yourself to process these feelings and seek support when needed. Talking to a counselor, joining a support group, or confiding in a trusted friend can provide a safe space to express and navigate your emotions.

Spiritually, this is a time to reconnect with your faith and find solace in God's presence. Spend time in prayer and meditation, seeking His guidance and comfort. Reflect on the ways God has been with you throughout your journey and trust that He will continue to be by your side.

Engage in activities that nurture your spirit, whether it's reading scripture, listening to worship music, or spending quiet moments in nature. These practices can help you find peace and strength as you move forward.

Remember, God is close to you, especially in moments of brokenness. He understands your pain and is there to support you through every step of your recovery. Lean on Him, and allow His love and grace to heal and restore you.

Prayer

Lord, thank You for being close to me in my times of need. Help me to recover mentally and spiritually as I move beyond cancer. Guide me in finding peace and strength in Your presence. Amen.

Reflection

- How can you support your mental and spiritual recovery during this time?

- What practices can help you feel closer to God and find solace in His presence?

- *What do I want to remember about my healing during this recovery process?*

A FUTURE BEYOND CANCER

"For I know the plans I have for you," declares the Lord, "plans to prosper you and not to harm you, plans to give you hope and a future."

— JEREMIAH 29:11

As I neared the end of my cancer treatment, a new sense of hope began to fill my heart. The journey had been long and arduous, but Jeremiah 29:11 reminded me that God had plans for my future—plans to give me hope and prosperity.

Looking ahead, I began to dream again. The thought of a future beyond cancer was both exhilarating and daunting. There were so many uncertainties, but I chose to trust in God's promises. He had carried me through the darkest valleys, and I believed He would guide me into a bright and hopeful future.

I started to set small goals for myself. Some were simple, like taking a walk every day or reconnecting with old friends. Others were more ambitious, like pursuing new career opportunities or traveling to places I had always wanted to visit. Each goal represented a step towards reclaiming my life and embracing the future God had in store for me.

Prayer became a crucial part of my planning process. I would spend quiet moments asking God to reveal His plans for me and to give me the courage to pursue them. Each prayer strengthened my faith and reassured me that I was not walking this path alone.

The journey beyond cancer is ongoing, but each day brings new opportunities and blessings. By trusting in God's plan and taking one step at a time, I am building a future filled with hope and joy.

Prayer

Lord, thank You for the promise of a hopeful future. As I move beyond cancer, guide me in setting goals and pursuing dreams that honor You. Strengthen my faith and fill me with courage as I embrace the plans You have for me. Amen.

Reflection

- What dreams and goals do you have for your future beyond cancer?
- How can you trust in God's plans and seek His guidance in pursuing them?

_____

_____

_____

_____

_____

YASMIN'S STORY - MANAGING LONG-TERM SIDE EFFECTS

"He gives strength to the weary and increases the power of the weak."

— ISAIAH 40:29

After completing her cancer treatment, Yasmin thought the hardest part was over. However, she soon realized that managing long-term side effects would be a new challenge. Fatigue, neuropathy, and other lingering issues made daily life difficult. But Isaiah 40:29 gave her strength: *"He gives strength to the weary and increases the power of the weak."*

Yasmin found comfort in her faith. Each day, she spent time in prayer, asking God for strength and guidance. She discovered that her spiritual practice not only provided emotional support but also helped her cope with physical discomfort.

In addition to prayer, Yasmin started exploring different holistic therapies. She tried gentle exercises like yoga and tai chi, which helped improve her mobility and reduce her neuropathy symptoms. She also experimented with aromatherapy and massage, finding that these practices helped alleviate her pain and promote relaxation.

Yasmin's doctors played a crucial role in managing her long-term side effects. Regular check-ups and open communication with her healthcare team ensured that she received the necessary treatments and adjustments to her care plan. This proactive approach made a significant difference in her quality of life.

Yasmin also leaned on her close-knit circle of friends and family. They provided practical help, such as assisting with household chores and accompanying her to medical appointments. Their support and encouragement gave her the strength to keep going, even on the toughest days.

Through her journey, Yasmin learned that managing long-term side effects required a combination of physical, emotional, and spiritual strategies. She found strength in her faith, her medical team, and the love of those around her.

Yasmin's story reminds us that while the battle with cancer may end, the journey of managing its effects continues. With God's strength and the support of others, you can navigate these challenges and find ways to thrive.

Prayer

Dear God, give me strength as I manage the long-term side effects of my treatment. Help me to find effective ways to cope and to lean on my support system. Thank You for increasing my power when I feel weak. Amen.

Reflection

- What long-term side effects are you managing, and how can you find strength in God's promises?

- How can you incorporate physical, emotional, and spiritual strategies into your daily routine?

REBUILDING RELATIONSHIPS

"A friend loves at all times, and a brother is born for a time of adversity."

— PROVERBS 17:17

As you transition to life beyond cancer, you may find that your relationships have changed. The journey through treatment can strain even the strongest bonds, but it also offers an opportunity to rebuild and strengthen those connections. Proverbs 17:17 reminds us that true friends and family are there for us in times of adversity.

Rebuilding relationships starts with open and honest communication. Share your experiences and feelings with your loved ones. Let them know how they can support you as you navigate this new chapter. Be willing to listen to their perspectives and understand how your journey has affected them as well.

It's important to acknowledge that both you and your loved ones may have changed. Give each other grace and patience as you adjust to these changes. Focus on the qualities that drew you together in the first place and build on them.

Forgiveness may also play a crucial role. There may be moments during your treatment when misunderstandings or conflicts arose. Now is the time to let go of past hurts and move forward with a spirit of forgiveness and reconciliation.

Reconnect with friends and family through shared activities and quality time. Whether it's a simple coffee date, a walk in the park, or a heartfelt conversation, these moments can help rebuild your bonds and create new, positive memories.

Remember that God is with you in this process. Pray for guidance and wisdom as you work to restore and strengthen your relationships. Trust that He is helping you to build connections that are deeper and more meaningful than ever before.

Prayer

Lord, thank You for the friends and family who have supported me through my journey. Help me to rebuild and strengthen these relationships with grace, patience, and love. Guide me in open communication and forgiveness. Amen.

Reflection

- How have your relationships changed during your cancer journey?
- What steps can you take to rebuild and strengthen your connections with loved ones?

_____

_____

_____

_____

RETURNING TO THE WORKPLACE

"Commit your work to the Lord, and your plans will be established."

— PROVERBS 16:3

Returning to the workplace after cancer treatment was a milestone I approached with a mixture of excitement and apprehension. Proverbs 16:3 became my guiding verse during this transition: *"Commit your work to the Lord, and your plans will be established."*

My first day back felt overwhelming. There were new faces, updated systems, and the ever-present fear of not being able to keep up. But I remembered that God was with me, and I chose to commit my work to Him. I started my day with prayer, asking for His strength and guidance.

The support from my colleagues made a significant difference. Many welcomed me back warmly, and I felt their genuine concern and encouragement. I shared my journey with them, which opened the door for deeper connections and understanding.

There were days when fatigue and side effects from treatment made work challenging. On those days, I leaned on God's promise and took things one step at a time. I also learned to listen to my body and give myself grace when I needed to rest.

As time went on, I found a new rhythm. My experiences had given me a fresh perspective on work and life. I was more patient, more appreciative of small achievements, and more compassionate towards others.

Returning to the workplace was not just about resuming my career; it was about embracing a new chapter with faith and resilience. Committing my work to the Lord helped me navigate this transition with confidence and peace.

Prayer

Lord, as I return to the workplace, help me to commit my work to You. Give me strength, guidance, and patience. Thank You for being with me every step of the way. Amen.

Reflection

- What fears or challenges do you face in returning to the workplace?

- How can you commit your work to the Lord and seek His guidance in this new chapter?

- *What do I want to remember about God's faithfulness and my personal growth as I step back into work?*

PHYSICAL REHABILITATION

"I can do all this through him who gives me strength."

— PHILIPPIANS 4:13

The journey of physical rehabilitation after cancer treatment can be daunting, but it is also a path to reclaiming your strength and vitality. Philippians 4:13 provides encouragement: *"I can do all this through him who gives me strength."*

As you embark on physical rehabilitation, picture yourself taking the first steps into a new chapter of recovery. Your body has endured so much, and now it's time to nurture it back to health. Imagine the feeling of stretching your limbs gently, the first tentative steps on a treadmill, or the calming flow of a yoga session. These activities are not just exercises; they are declarations of your resilience.

Each morning, you may find yourself stretching a little further or walking a bit longer. Feel the strength gradually returning to your muscles, the improvement in your balance, and the increase in your stamina. Celebrate these small victories, for each one is a testament to your determination and God's sustaining power.

On difficult days, when fatigue and pain seem overwhelming, remember to listen to your body and give yourself grace. Rest is as much a part of rehabilitation as activity. Visualize God's comforting presence beside you, holding you up when you feel weak. Pray for His strength and perseverance, and let His love be the balm for your weary soul.

Incorporate mindfulness into your routine. Spend a few moments each day in prayer and meditation, inviting God's peace to fill your heart. Picture yourself enveloped in His comforting embrace, His strength flowing through you, empowering each movement.

Your support system plays a crucial role in this journey. Lean on friends, family, and healthcare professionals who can offer encouragement and practical assistance. Imagine their smiles, their words of support, and their hands ready to help you as you rebuild your strength.

Remember, you are not alone. God is with you, providing the strength you need to overcome each hurdle. Trust in His power and continue to move forward with faith and determination.

Prayer

Lord, give me strength and patience as I work towards physical rehabilitation. Help me to celebrate the small victories and to trust in Your power to guide me through this journey. Thank You for being my source of strength. Amen.

Reflection

- What small steps can you take today towards your physical rehabilitation?

- How can you incorporate prayer and meditation into your rehabilitation routine?

CELEBRATING SURVIVORSHIP

"Give thanks to the Lord, for he is good; his love endures forever."

— PSALM 107:1

Congratulations, warrior. You've made it through the storm, and now you stand on the other side as a survivor. Psalm 107:1 captures the depth of gratitude you might feel: *"Give thanks to the Lord, for he is good; his love endures forever."*

Reaching this milestone is a testament to your strength and resilience. You've fought hard, endured countless challenges, and emerged victorious. Whether your journey was marked by moments of doubt or unwavering faith, you've proven that you are strong and capable. You are a survivor.

As you reflect on your journey, take a moment to celebrate the battles you've won and the courage you've shown. Acknowledge the physical, emotional, and spiritual growth that has taken place. You've discovered new strengths and depths within yourself that you might not have known existed.

Whatever the future holds, know that you are equipped to face it. If there are lingering side effects or ongoing treatments, remember that you have already come so far. Trust in God's continuous presence and support. His love endures forever, and He will guide you through every new challenge.

Consider how you can give back and share your story. Your journey can be a beacon of hope for others who are walking a similar path. Whether it's through volunteering, speaking at support groups, or simply offering a listening ear to a fellow survivor, your experiences can provide strength and encouragement to others.

Celebrate the small moments and the big milestones. Embrace the joy of everyday life and the beauty of simple pleasures. Each day is a gift, a testament to your perseverance and God's faithfulness.

You are not just a survivor; you are a thriver. You have faced adversity and emerged stronger. Continue to lean on your faith, and remember that God's love and goodness are with you always.

Prayer

Lord, thank You for carrying me through my journey. Help me to celebrate my survivorship with gratitude and to share my story to inspire and support others. Thank You for Your enduring love and faithfulness. Amen.

Reflection

- How can you celebrate your survivorship and acknowledge the battles you've won?

- In what ways can you give back and offer hope to others on similar journeys?

DATE

S M T W T F S

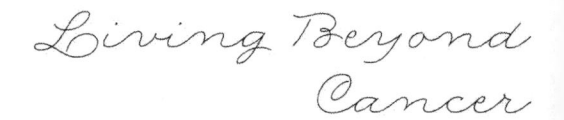

Living Beyond Cancer

TRY NEW THINGS

Think of three new activities or experiences you've always wanted to try.

New Activity 1	
New Activity 2	
New Activity 3	

SHARE YOUR STORY

Consider sharing your journey with others, whether through a support group, a blog, or a conversation with a friend.

How does sharing your story help you reflect on your journey?

_____
_____
_____
_____
_____
_____
_____
_____
_____

SET NEW GOALS

Think about what you want to achieve in this new chapter of your life. Set your new goals and the first step toward each one:

As you move forward, embrace new experiences, stay connected, and appreciate how far you've come.

PASS ON THE BLESSINGS

"Therefore encourage one another and build each other up, just as in fact you are doing."

— 1 THESSALONIANS 5:11

As you come to the end of this devotional, you carry with you a wealth of strength, hope, and inspiration that has helped you through your journey with cancer. Now, it's time to share your experiences and guide others to find the same comfort and support.

By leaving your honest opinion of this book on Amazon, you'll show other women facing cancer where they can find the encouragement and solace they need. Your review can make a real difference in helping them feel less alone and more uplifted during this challenging time.

Thank you for your help. The journey through cancer is made lighter when we share our stories and support one another – and you're helping us to do just that.

Scan below to leave your review on Amazon.

[Insert QR Code]

Your review is not just feedback; it's a gift of hope and encouragement for other women on this path. Thank you for being a part of this community sharing the strength and love that unites us. May God bless you with peace and healing, and may your story be a light for others.

With heartfelt gratitude,

Biblical Teachings

AND SO, THE JOURNEY CONTINUES...

You've come so far on this journey with such courage and grace. Whether stepping into a new chapter post-treatment, living in remission, or finding strength in a different phase, you have faced this path with remarkable resilience. This journey doesn't end here; it continues to unfold, bringing new experiences and growth.

As you move forward, may you feel the deep peace that comes from knowing God walks with you every step of the way. The lessons and reflections you've encountered here are meant to stay with you, offering comfort and guidance whenever needed. Let these words remind you that you are never alone and that hope and love surround you.

You have a beautiful story, one that is filled with bravery, faith, and the love of those who care for you. Sharing your experiences can be a light for others on similar paths, offering them hope and encouragement. Your strength and compassion are powerful; your story can touch many hearts.

We are so grateful to have been part of your journey through this devotional. It has been a privilege to offer words of support and to

AND SO, THE JOURNEY CONTINUES...

stand with you in prayer. Please remember that you are deeply loved and cherished by those around you and by God.

As you look ahead, know that the future holds many moments of joy and peace. Embrace each day confidently, trusting in God's loving plan for you. Your story is still unfolding, and many beautiful and fulfilling moments will come. May you continue to find strength, comfort, and hope in God's love, now and always.

With warmest wishes and prayers,

The team at Biblical Teachings

Made in the USA
Columbia, SC
06 April 2025